Obese – No More

How I lost More than 90 Kg (198 lbs)

By Corrie Lamprecht

Thank you for considering this Book.

I trust this book will be a great help in achieving your dreams to a happy and healthy life.

Thank you for your support.

Knowledge comes from Understanding;

Understanding is due to Knowledge;

The one feeds on the other.

Corrie Lamprecht (2015)

A perfect healthy body; is a balanced body.

If the balance is heavy on one side;

You need to put more weight on the other side;

BUT do not tip the scale over.

Corrie Lamprecht (2007)

IN THE BODY - NOTHING WORKS IN ISOLATION.

Disclaimer.

This book is not written to and does not provide medical advice, professional diagnosis, opinion, treatment or services to you or to any other individual. I, the author, and any other person who might be involved with this book does not claim ourselves to be a medical professional. Neither do we give any guarantees of anything – other than my own personal experience in this book.

At best, that which is written in this book may be seen as suggestions for you and your doctor to research and provide general information for educational purposes only. This is my life story and based on how I changed my life in the months before writing this book. If you decide to embark on your own experiments or to follow those that I did – it is entirely at your own wish, your own risk and on your own responsibility. Nobody else can be held responsible, neither does anybody accept any responsibility for your action in relation to anything written or stated in this book.

Neither the Author or any other person involved with this book, or any references to any other information piece, are liable or responsible for any advice, course of treatment, diagnosis or any other information, reference, services or product you obtain through this book or any related sites.

For safety, I would suggest you see a medical practitioner before, during and after your (or any) weight loss program.

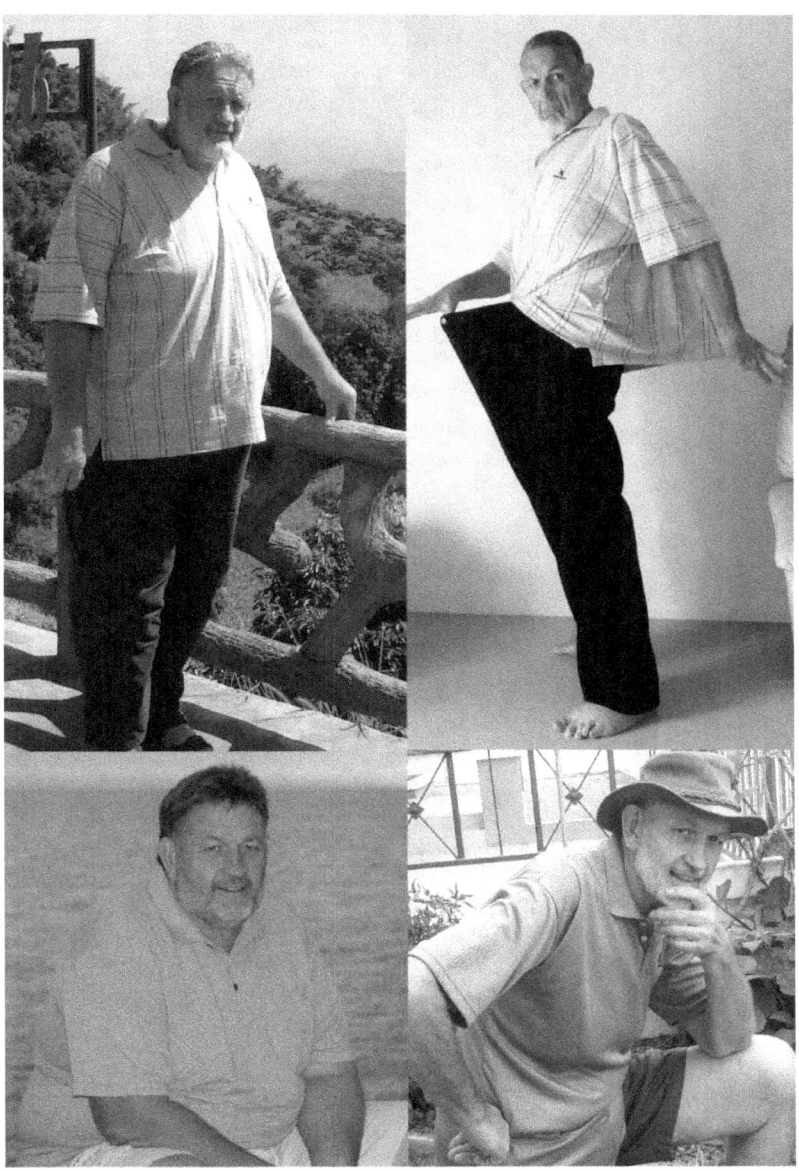

A few before and current photos. The blue polo shirt on top is the same one, taken exactly 12 months apart. The pants however is size 56" (Dating back to 2002) while my top size was 66" – those unfortunately disposed of few months ago.

Index.

Disclaimer. .... - 4 -

Index. .... - 6 -

About this book... - 7 -

Introduction. .... - 10 -

The Secret Formula for Losing Weight. .... - 18 -

Chapter 1 - My Story. .... - 24 -

Chapter 2 - Weight Loss. .... - 45 -

Chapter 3 - Potato Only Diet.. - 85 -

Chapter 4 - One Meal A Day. .... - 94 -

Chapter 5 - High Fat Diet & Ketosis. .... - 97 -

Chapter 6 - Problems. .... - 103 -

Chapter 7 - My Weight Loss Medicine. .... - 135 -

Chapter 8 - An Open Letter to myself. .... - 150 -

Chapter 9 - Staying slim and healthy. .... - 154 -

Chapter 10 - Additional Information. .... - 155 -

Chapter 11 - External Information.. - 166 -

About this book.

I started gaining weight nine months before I was born. By the time I saw the light of life, I was already an oversized baby. The gaining of weight relentlessly went on and upwards until I was 57 years old. Regardless how hard I tried, how many this or that diet programs I did through my life, the loss of weight was just not possible. Even going on fasting for three or four days with only water did not had me lose weight, a kilogram or so which was basically just water – diuretic. Then, at 57 years of age, for the first time in my life I lost a bit of weight. It was not until I was 59 that many things came together and I could really lose a lot of weight.

This book is not so much for people who want just another series of secret recipes. I may make videos about my cooking, and link to other videos of the same which I found very helpful. To keep updated you might wish to subscribe to my website, YouTube Channel and/or Facebook page. See last pages of this book for links.

Neither is this book for those who wants to lose a couple of pounds or kg. Certainly you will learn some good ideas, and it can help you to lose those few kilograms of weight. All you need to do for a few kilograms of weight loss is to cut out all forms of sugar and grain for a short period of time; that is very easy. You will not find secret formulae for small weight loss in this book.

This is my story for those who has a life long struggle with excessive weight.

This book will be especially valuable for those who realize their scale reading are getting relentlessly higher and they suffer to get weight under control.

Here is one enlightening point: The same problems that makes you gaining weight, becoming fat – that same is usually also responsible for a myriad of other health issues. Here I am not only talking of blood and heart; but diabetes, backache, bone problems, brain issues like Alzheimer's, thyroid issues, and even the big Cancer.

It is not a one month bang course, this is about many months, even a year or two of dedication about getting your own body fixed and yourself on the path of health for prolonged life. This book is aimed to give a little better information and to explain many issues which might be the underlying foundation of your problems – as it was mine. But, you will need to put in a lot of effort to learn.

I share not only the good success story; but I will also talk about the mistake(s) I made.

Funny enough, I will not push you on exercise – just as I did not push myself to exhaustion in an expensive gym either. You will not need a food scale, you will not follow strict dietary rules . . . well, maybe a few easy ones.

This might not be the same situation for everyone. Therefore, much of the material in this book is about understanding the issue behind excess weight and your own body; and how to fix that.

If you are obese, or super obese or like I was 'morbidly obese' then this book might solve your lifelong quest for a better looking, better feeling and a hell of a lot healthier you.

Being overweight is often also the cause for other ailments, some even serious. Some of these related issues will be clear to you after reading this book and cross checking the information. Surprising how much better my general health became after I started on this road – even before losing much weight. There are some 'secrets' – for mysterious reasons hidden from general public; maybe financial reasons?

I trust this writing is going to help many people lose their extra unwanted baggage; and live a more enjoyable life – as I do now.

I had a difficult issue with chronology in this book. That mostly because the human body is a great network of bio-chemical processes, where the one affects the other. Thus, as you read you will have questions. Please do read the book through at least once, to see later sections which might have a bounce-back effect to a piece you read earlier. Then you can read it again and take notes.

A story:

Two old men sit on a bench, talking about hunting wild ducks. Each has a shotgun and a basket. One of them has two freshly cleaned ducks ready for cooking in it. The other is a very professional hunter, he knows everything; but his basket is empty. Both tell you a slightly different story about the best way to hunt ducks. Who would you believe?

Introduction.

A hefty 187.6 Kg is the only provable recorded number I have, but I was a few kilograms higher. I remember the tightness of my clothes; before the hospital got the new scales. At the top, my weight was probably around 200 Kg (440 pounds). By that time, even my legs gave in and standing or walking became a painful activity.

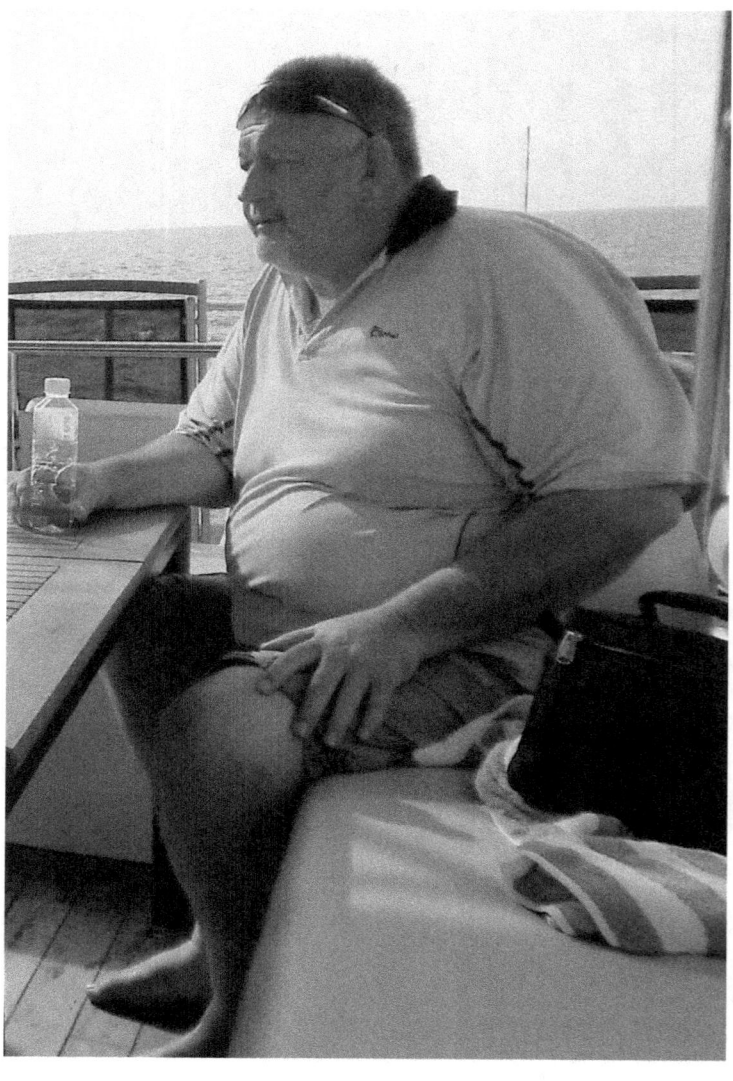

With great difficulty and very hard work over a period of two years I finally succeeded in bringing my weight down to the low of 165 kg. That was where I got stuck again. Very hard work to just maintain my weight and then the worst news from my bedroom scale. Weight going upwards again. 166, 167, desperation sets in, stop eating, 168, 169, fasting, 170, 171, WTF, I can't stand this, why is it not going down, 172 seriously hard exercise routines, minimum eating, 173, 174, relentless up. In May 2016 I was back at 174.8 kg.

Then I learned something new - and I did that something. In 10 months my weight dropped from 174 .8 kg (385 lbs) right down to the current 98 Kg (216 lbs). That loss of 77 Kg is more than most people should weigh in total.

I will share with you some things nobody, not even those closest to me, knew about. One early morning, I sat half way up on the stairs to my own first floor office crying; because I could not get up the stairs.

Those recent funny days when I come across people that knew me as Big Corrie – and their astonished faces when they finally recognise the slimmer me. The day in the Mall when I walk right past my ex-girlfriend of nine years and she did not recognise me! Hey, that day when my daughter in law saw me on the boat … it took her a while to add 'the familiar posture' and me together as Corrie.

I invite you to learn how the marvellous refinery factory of your body works. I wish this book to be a motivation and maybe some ideas to help people like the Old me to finally unwrap their true hidden self.

What I am presenting in this book is not a Scientific Paper, neither just another "Diet Book". I wrote about my experience, what I learned and how I finally lost a total of over 90 Kg of fat. Now my struggle is a bit easier – not to lose more!

REMEMBER: I was there, I did it. This is my real physical experience. I have the loose skin as medals to prove it!

WARNING: What I finally did was in true desperation, it worked for me. But it might be dangerous. This is my story; I do not recommend nor instruct nor suggest any person to do the same. Whatever you do – you and YOU ALONE can, will and should make a decision. Go and learn more, follow up on the scenarios I will talk about. Things like the One Meal a Day concept, pH controls, the foods, the minerals … etc.

Is it not funny that mainstream medical profession fails in the most basic of application to make people healthier? Use this knowledge to gain more understanding. It is amazing how much we learn through our lives, about our school education, our college, universities, and our jobs. How to be a parent and how to make or save money. Yet, of the one most important thing in our lives – most people know and understand so little, often most people knows nothing at all;

Your own body.

That is most precious possession you will ever have in all of your living existence.

I do not say you need to know as much as a medical doctor or pathologist, though it would definitely be an advantage to your own self. As someone told me a while back "*I do not need to know all these things of my body. When I get sick, I go to a doctor or the hospital. They studied it all in great details and can take care of it.*"

Well Mr K might have been right in his own mind. But I think he was wrong. In the historical times of some Asian regions (and still in some smaller villages) this was working perfectly. You could absolutely trust the village doctor to do the best for every person living there. See, in those times and locale the health practitioner was only remunerated while everybody in the village is healthy. The moment somebody gets sick, his/her income or remuneration seized until everybody is healthy again. If somebody dies, besides the reason of old age, then there was even an extended period of nothing to the health practitioner. This is not so anymore.

Here is something you MUST understand, it is critical to know. Today every action of just about everybody in the whole world is about making money. The health profession is not excluded. Yes, there are many true good hearted health practitioners whose wish is to heal people. Normally you may find them not too wealthy. Often they are of the Alternative medicine camp.

The general medical profession, from doctor, through hospital and supported by the massive Pharmaceutical companies and their millions of pharmacies – they are ALL about making money. They never issue an annual report on how many people they healed. The annual reports are only about how much income they generated and what the dividends payable to their shareholders are. It is about making money. Healthy people do not buy their products! Healthy people do not generate income for Pharma, doctor or hospital. Thus the pure plain logic is that they need you to feel good, but come back for more … of whatever medicines they want to stuff down your throat. And that is only applicable while you have some coloured bank papers in your wallet.

Sorry, I can rant for hours around this issue. Better move on, but let me place one final statement:

DO NOT trust your medical advisor blindly. Not any doctor, pharmacist, hospital, or advisor – and do not trust what I wrote here either. Please DO your own research, always double check. Get a second and even a third opinion. After all, it is only your health and your life in your own hands.

We wrongly learned that losing weight is all about diet and exercise. That is probably true for many people, but it is not always the dominant factor. Why can some people eat anything they want in any quantity they want – yet they are thin? Without strenuous exercises. Why did my grandparents, in South Africa, ate the worst kind of fatty meat, potato, eggs, bacon, wheat, corn, sweet preserved fruits, jelly and whatever is today considered unhealthy - every day in big portions – yet they were not obese and lived beyond 90 years of age?

There is something amiss here. Why is it that in this modern world, we see annual growth in the percentage of obese people, everywhere? The good old USA leads the way with 68% overweight; and 36% of the total population falling in the category 'Obese' or higher. Why do we fail to lose weight and keep it off our bodies?

I went on a search and research. I did a lot of things and finally I achieved a huge success. I lost a total of 90 Kilograms. AND NOT PICKING IT UP AGAIN.

Besides the losing of weight, there are lots of pointers which may lead you to an easily achievable healthy lifestyle.

I have been trying to lose weight for more than 40 years. Many different kinds of diets, options, and methods. Yet, I failed attempt after attempt. But I also got more and more desperate in this last few years when my legs gave in to such extend that walking became a major laborious task. My blood pressure were extreme 184/120/60. My heartbeat was irregular, legs swelling up from water retention and many more issues.

I pulled out all my Anatomy and Physiology books and I went through the internet searching and absorbing information like a sponge. Is it not amazing! Some Medical 'educated' will tell you that you should stop eating grain – another say no you have to eat only grain. Or stop eating all forms of meat, another says eat fatty meat. Don't drink fruit juices – drink fruit juices. Drink 10 glasses of warm water, do not consume any salt . . . What a lot of crap. But they all sell you pills and capsules with a scalpel ready behind their back to cut you open. One can only feel lost, like a Roman Gladiator being forced between two armed columns of soldiers to slaughter. There you go – can't go left, can't go right – if you go straight you will gain more weight and die a crippled sick person. Going back is not possible – the time has passed.

I got tired of all this bullshit. Then I started thinking. Fortunately I did travel quite a bit around the world. I have been in most Asian countries, many in Africa and some in Europe. America I did not visit myself, but one can see enough of them on TV. I did notice a remarkable fact.

The less developed countries have thin people, the more the country is 'developed' the weightier are the people. It is not because they eat less; it is because of what they eat. Ahh, Singapore, Hong Kong – and my home for this past 17 years – Thailand. Strange to notice in Thailand the people are getting more and more obese – BUT only in the bigger cities and the areas where they are commonly in contact with European foreigners like Bangkok, Pattaya and Phuket. In neighbouring Cambodia, Laos and Myanmar the same genetic people are in a much healthier proportion.

Hey, here is a secret. Genetics has absolutely nothing to do with your weight. Period. Read this line again.

Now let us see what the main diets of the Thai are; at least those that are not overweight. They eat lots of rice. But rice is an empty nutrient depleted grain, starch is not really a good nutritious food source. Did you know they were using rice powder to make paper in ancient China? Secondary they eat lots of Chicken, Pork and Fish in that order. The pork, well that is really something between fatty and extremely fat. The chickens are mostly deep fried in palm oil. The fish, well if they are close to the sea they can get quite a bit of marine fish. More inland they eat mostly farmed fish – Tilapia and catfish. And then there are the prawns, lots of prawns.

Hey what is wrong with this protein part of their diets? It is all against what I learned years ago about good food and bad food. Did I mention that most – probably 70% - of all the Thai protein food is deep fried in oil? So it is very unhealthy. But nice. It is supposed to make you very unhealthy; and obese.

On top of this, the Thai people are eating a lot of greens, herbs – and let us not forget the spices, especially various chillies. Spices WOW, those are deadly for you because your body can not easily dispose of it. Well, that is what I was wrongly educated to believe.

Go into the big cities and farang (European Foreigner) areas and you immediately find their diets changed and the general cross cut of people are somewhere between overweight and obese. Why? Because they started eating wrong. Wrong food, wrong combinations – and they consume a LOT more sugar. Oh, the sugar. There you find a lovely drink next to the road. They take a sugar cane, squeeze it through a press, all the pure sugar juice into a little plastic bag filled with ice – Sugar sweet drink. Grrr.

In earlier times the Thai people did love their sweet; but that was from pure natural honey.

Lately, I will say the last 10 years or so, many a school has a 7-Eleven just around the corner. And in those cases you find the bigger (horizontal measure) of kids. In the more rural areas, where the population does not justify a 7-Eleven yet, you find ladies cooking Thai food for the kids just outside the gates. By all dietician measure, extremely fatty, oily, unhealthy foods. At least according to dietary standards. Hey, those kids are so healthy, energetic and perfect body proportions.

So what is it with 7-Eleven? I took a careful look and will tell you there is just about nothing in a 7-Eleven that does not have a large portion of sugar. I mean even the bread, rolls, cold meats, nuts, noodle soup cups, yoghurt, drinks . . . just about everything is stuffed with sugar. Those few items that might not have lots of sugar, are stuffed with MSG for preservation . . . Hmm, it does not stop there. Go to any of the big supermarkets, here we have Robinson, Tesco Lotus, Tops and Big-C, and try to find diet friendly foods anywhere except the vegetables section. In some big centres you may find a very small (read less than 1% floor space) with 'Healthy foods' – and those are horrifically expensive. I can only presume the same is valid all over the modern Western World. Sugar, sugar, sugar.

I wonder why less processed flour is more expensive? Or why is a packet of rice with the shells still on double the price of the highly refined one?

The sugar is really bad, but sugar with anything else in combination is immediately ten times worse. Wherever you find the American giants like MacDonald's, Dunking Doughnuts, Kentucky Fried Chicken – you find the general cross cut population is growing . . . in width and weight.

- The Secret Formula!

Yes, right here and right now I will tell you the whole secret. Only five steps. Everything I did to lose weight. You can jump in and do the same, if you wish. This is a simple concept, but be warned. You do need to understand what will happen, why it happens – and maybe why it may not work in your body. Above all, you need to be aware of the progress, symptoms and when things might go the wrong way. Else, you WILL fail.

Step 1: Stop hungry feelings and eat less.

Step 2: Raise digestive system pH.

Step 3: Raise blood / cellular pH.

Step 4: Eat fatty foods, no carbohydrates.

Step 5: Watch the scale.

- So, what is this book about?

1. What definitely NOT to eat.
2. Re-Teach your body.
3. Learn to listen to your body.
4. Control of pH and minerals.
5. A new you; a healthier life.
6. It is NOT a strict diet.
7. It is NOT hard gym sweating exercise.

The Secret Formula for Losing Weight.

What diet book is ever written without these words? Thus I have to say it, else nobody may consider buying my book, right? Now let me tell you in very short what the secret of this whole 'system' is. But, keep in mind that these are just headlines. Unless you understand your own body and know what to expect when it happens – these secrets are just like the Big Hoaxes of the world. Empty wind.

- The Biggest Secret.

Some people are fat, others are thin; there is a common joke from the fatter people against the thinner people. 'We are able to survive for longer without food.' In fact, that is exactly true. It is a somewhat misconception that fat is stored energy. The building up of fat in the body is all about SURVIVAL. The main source of energy for the body is from sugars.

BUT; this is one little fact you have to permanently imprint into your mind. All the sugars in your blood, if dried and lumped together will not exceed a heaped spoon of volume. Yet, that is what your body requires for a normal active life of about three whole days. Your body needs sugar to live but before you jump to the candy store; there is an issue of how much. Your body needs about 5 to 6 grams of sugar per day – that is just about a teaspoon. And, that includes all forms of sugar – glucose, sucrose, fructose, etc. Anything more than this . . . becomes fat.

"Fat is a survival gland that protects against the starvation of sugar. It means that fat is the back-up against the depletion of sugar. Your body will not survive for longer than 72 hours without fat. That is why your body stores fat." Dr Eric Berg.

1. You should learn to understand your own body and learn communicating with your own body. See the symptoms of things that are happening before they happen. Although I can't possibly present all and everything related in this book, I will cover the few critical basic symptoms with relation to this weight loss program.

2. Allow your body to balance itself again.

3. Stop all sugars in your food. Do not eat any added sugar anywhere, anytime. Dead STOP.

4. Drink lots of pure healthy balanced water – at least 1.5 litre per day.

5. Eat meat (fatty meat) and other types of fat like avocado, real butter, certain cooking oils, nuts, etc. Yip, that is true but I will explain later. Oh yes, eat potatoes, plenty of them - sometimes. I guess this is a shocker. But if you are a strict vegetarian then do not fear, you can substitute other proteins for the meat part.

6. Exercise? Sweating gym? Nope, not now and not until you reached your desired weight – then YES. But until that stage, just a bit of walking and stretching routines. You will not even breathe strong. Let us be honest, if you are morbidly obese the word exercise is the last thing you want to hear about. You know and I know just walking a few meters takes a huge effort. Imagine a gym full of dancing, hopping weight pushing pretty bodies all around you. That only compares to a horror movie; and depression.

7. The biggest secret? Eat less times per day, eat less food per day and eat a lot more nutritious food per day. With this you will get the appetite and hormones in your body under control; and weight will drop.

8. Ahh, then the second true BIG secret. Change your body acidity or alkalinity. Change what you eat and how you eat. Now this sounds easy. Hey, pop a spoon of Baking Soda in a bottle of water three times a day and whoooaaa weight gone. Nope, this is the most critical part but this requires for you to understand what will happen and why it happens; and the risks.

9. There is one easy method, many went for it. I choose to say never. You go to a medical specialist and let them cut out those you should not have. One operation that does help many people today is where the cut your stomach smaller and make a bypass. It is expensive and a number of people (UK is around 12%) who did such drastic steps, never woke up afterwards. Cutting on my body is never an option. Many of those who had a great success, the weight returned three or four years later.

So, let us get on with the fun stuff. Getting to learn about this wonderful bio-chemical factory we call our own personal body; and how to bring our hidden self to the front again.

All I can say is I HAVE DONE IT – after many years of unbelievable struggle, I am down to a size that does not make people turn their heads behind my back anymore. Walking into a place full of people does not result in a stunned silence. I do not get the question "How much do you weigh?" anymore. The Thai people can be unbelievably blunt, sometimes. I believe you can dig your better looking self out from amongst all those blabber. In a very natural way. Lose a lot of weight.

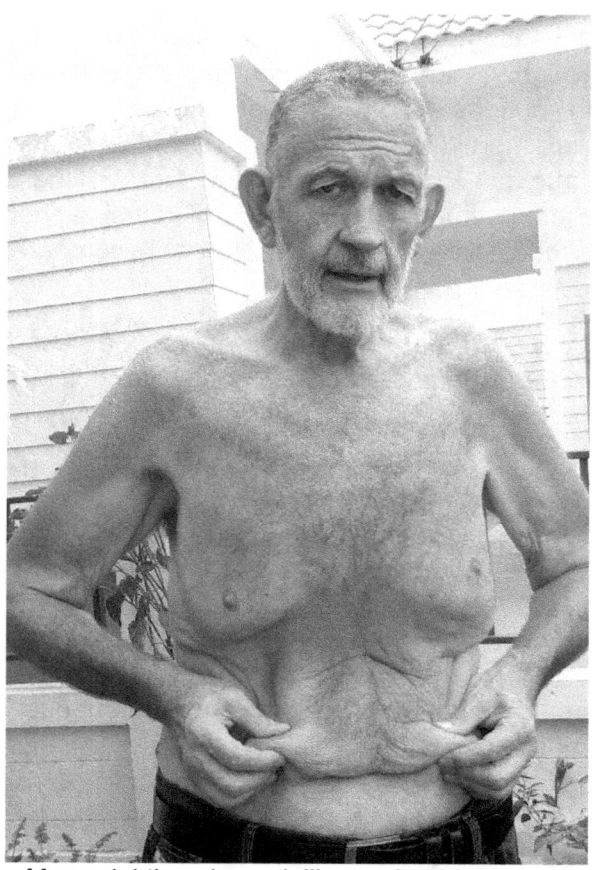

My unsightly ugly medallions – but I have is as proof that I did something unique.

Oh, yes there is however one thing that is not too pleasant, or should I say pretty? That is what is called 'Loose skin'. Tell you it is not always a pretty sight; especially if you are 60-year-old man like me. But I am working on that, if I succeed there will be a new book. However, for now, since I am such a positive person – I look, I see and I am proud. That loose skin is my medallion. It is the proof that I had successfully done something very few people in this world could achieve.

I do believe there is going to be some ways of coping and reducing this, off course – the younger you are, the more likely you can get it to go away and remain with a fairly good tighter skin.

I have lost the 90% extra deadly weight that was loaded inside my precious body. Let me rephrase this; I am half the size I used to be.

- The magnificent YOU.

The miracle of life, the wonders of our creation. Just imagine two little microscopic things comes together and then they blended, forms a heliacal DNA string and then you started to be formed. One cell, two cells, four cells, until the estimated 33 trillion cells that you are today. Yet, regardless of all these, you are just a bunch of minute cells that work together. You are like a big Bio-Chemical factory – in unison working together to be the unique you.

Your body is in effect a chemical plant, not only biological, but full blown chemical. As you find in any such, there are laboratories, machinery, processes, control rooms, pumps, filters, pipes, valves, electrical systems, et al. Yes, indeed you have exactly the same as a major factory. An interesting thing is that sometimes your body can manufacture things inside it which even factories cannot do to this day!

It is only by beginning to understand how our bodies actually works – that we can control our health and extend our longevity. I have absolute no intend to teach you the medical anatomical way of understanding, there are plenty of other sources where you can learn this. I am going to share with you the very basic outline of how and what happens in your body by a different means, that of a Bio-Chemical Refinery; and only from the perspective of our weight control.

Most often, this is one of the aspects never understood in the mainstream, never taught in universities. Let me give you one example.

We go for a general check-up and blood test. Such blood test then indicates we have a low level of Iron. Iron is an important element required in our blood and wonderful bodies. So the doctors prescribe iron tablets to us. Pure logical, yes? In truth it is not correct. See, our body does not like to receive a finished product from which it has to make a finished product! Our bodies often likes to make their own materials, to its own standards – and then use that. The underlying problem is that we might have a stomach acidity problem, resulting from a magnesium deficiency – and that leads to the body failing to absorb iron. The interesting thing is that for our Magnesium levels to be increased we need to consume Sodium. The body will use that Sodium to make the required Magnesium. But; the conditions inside the body must be right, else the process will fail.

This funny requirement and process in the body has a very curious title: Biological Transmutation.

Ever since our ancient times, we humans and our Alien Gods, tried to make Gold from other elements. Just read about all the alchemists dreaming of this magical processes during this past few millennia. To this day, it is the big quest in the mind of many a chemist, though not only in relation to gold.

We have small and big and massive particle colliders; build with the purpose of changing one element into another by collision at extreme speed, temperatures and pressures. And they have been quite successful. During the past decade or so at least 8 new minerals have been added to our updated periodic table of elements, mostly heavier metals.

The second method in which one element is transmuted into another is by means of radioactivity, this process is also applied by nature. I may write more about radioactive transmutation later in a book about cancer.

The third, and certainly the most interesting, is the Biological Transmutation of elements and minerals. This is the most critically important one for ALL living creatures, including our lovely bodies. This is what we need to understand. Yet, it is the least known process in our academic world. Something I fail to understand. Quite astonishing that in the medical and scientific communities this is a very controversial issue. The failure of this fraction in chemistry is one of the reasons why the living creatures on this earth is getting more and more sick by the day.

A few of the more common known biological transmutations in the body are: calcium to magnesium, sodium to potassium, calcium to potassium and sodium to magnesium. Did you notice, the body uses either Sodium or Calcium and then itself will make either Magnesium or Potassium as required? Really a fascinating body we have. How about Vitamin-C + Sunshine = Vitamin-D.

Just in the passing by, there is one other vitamin that is usually produced by our own bodies. It has been found that this Vitamin-K2 is of critical importance in blood clotting and other liver related issues. Yet, trying to find more information one runs into statements like; *"The precise contribution of the bacterially synthesized menaquinone to overall vitamin K requirements in man is unknown."*

Chapter 1 - My Story.

A baby boy was born on 4th December 1956 in Vanderbijlpark, South Africa. Little Corrie was a whopping 9 pounds and 4 ounces. It was an hour or so before the sunrise of that day. Right from that moment, when he was already a bit bigger than the normal, he started gaining weight. Just like any normal kid, but a little bit faster. Fortunately, for most of his life, he was not obese – just overweight. "Big body type, big bones" they said.

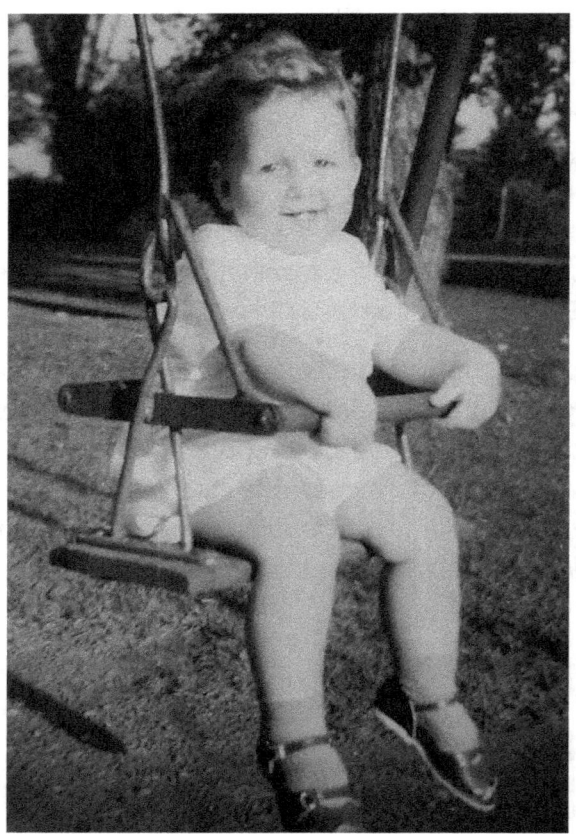

About one year of age.

Throughout his school days he was taller than all his classmates, and a bit on the heavier side too. A bit different from the usual, little Corrie was reasonably strong. Moving from Primary School to High School there is an initiation period. Corrie was mostly considered as either too big or older group, so he was saved the worst of humiliations. At one stage there were a group of some five or six senior kids trying to get him into a cold bath; but they could not hold him. Might have had something to do with the steel tips hand-me-down factory worker shoes from his father. Or it might have been because at that 13-year age he was already over 65 kg of weight.

Corrie dreamed of being a great boxer, fortunately his father blocked him from that. Just imagine what all the hitting on his head would have done to his poor brains. Thus, he took up Amateur Wrestling and Karate at the age of 15 years. When he started wrestling, his weight was 82 Kg and he was in the Heavy Weight section, only for just over a year. By 17 years of age he joined the South African Police force (SAP). During the one-year training Corrie was wrestling in the weight group Extra Heavy (Above 110 Kg). He was the second biggest student amongst the slight over 1,200 recruits for that year.

By the end of the SAP training year, reasonably fit and all, the weight of Corrie was around 120 Kg. It remained fairly steady between 120 kg and 130 kg for a few years. As young adult his height was 198 cm. Thus not looking obese, but not thin either. When he started to buy his own clothes (at 17 years of age), the shirts were of size XXL and pants around 120 cm (48 inch).

Regardless of fitness, exercises and even during a sting in the Youth outreach of the Church for two years when there was regular fasting of two to five days with only water to drink – Corrie never lost a single kilogram of weight. Even to him, this was a fascinating story.

At the age of 39 he was in a relationship with a pretty Jewish girl. Lynda tried her absolute best to reduce the size of Corrie by whatever means. There were months of early morning workouts, every single day, under supervision in the gym. Months of Weight Watchers and Weigh Less meetings and carefully measured diets, tablets, shakes, drinks and whatever. Corrie even stayed with Lynda and never could she find him cheating on his exercise nor diet – because he did not. He was just as serious to try and bring his weight down from the 138 Kg to somewhere under 110 Kg. Lynda, weight watchers and the personal trainers could not get his weight down, whatever they did.

Life went by, Corrie gave up on weight control and just went on with living. It was difficult enough to earn money anyway. By the change of the millennium he moved to Thailand and started a gemstone cutting factory. That followed by a short stint in the Middle east of about 18 months and then back to Thailand where he finally started a boat building factory in 2004.

What his weight was at that stage he does not know. It was still the era of dial-scales and they mostly did not go above 126 Kg anyway. But what he does know is that his shirts were of 4XL size and jeans were 56 inch. He still had some of these in storage when he lost weight in 2016.

As it was in Thailand, he needed to renew his work permit every year. A procedure that usually requires a medical certificate. It did not really bother anybody because the hospital where he went had a scale to weigh people – but the maximum weight that could measure was 160 Kg. So that was recorded as such on the hospital record.

The issue was blood pressure. On a few occasions the nurses did not want to record the blood pressure, because it was too high. Corrie usually said it was because of stress, test again after few minutes. Out the door he went, down the street to a pharmacy and buy a packet of anti-high blood pressure tablets. Popped two, take a long fast walk and back to the hospital "Measure again".

So what was the high blood pressure? Before tablets, it was usually around 185 Systole, 120 Diastole with a pulse rate of 65. After the tiring street stint, it usually came down to around 160/110/72 – which was somewhat more acceptable. Now, Corrie did know the problems, after all he did study medicine and a great deal about anatomy and physiology. A good normal blood pressure is around 120/80/60. However, the pressure for financial survival made all of these fade in the mist – until the next year December when he needed to go for Medical Certificate again.

Corrie had his office in the boat factory on the first floor. He usually went to office in early morning and worked until late night, mostly 14 to 16 hours every day. In 2010 he started developing severe pains and failure of the left knee and right hip. To such extend that normal walking was not possible anymore. Gout was the convenient excuse. His son made him a special super strong set of crutches from stainless steel. Still, getting up the stairs was extremely difficult. Listen, even getting up from bed or a chair was a major issue for him. Going to the office in the early morning was just as well, because he would not be seen by the workers struggling to get up the stairs. He often had to sit down on the stair and lift himself up step-by-step on his bums.

As if that was not enough, he also had a big problem in the lungs. The only way he could get through the days were by sucking additional oxygen from a tank. One green tank next to his bed, one in the car and two in the office. Went to have his lungs checked, the medicals find he has cancer in the lower bronchial tube, right at the split to the left and right lungs. There was nothing they could do – but for chemotherapy, which the doctor stated might not work. He suspects it was a residue from the times when he was working in the Uranium Refinery at Hartebeestpoort mine in South Africa. He always had a bronchial infection two or three times per year. Corrie declined the chemo because he did not think it will help, do not want to go through that issue and sufferings; and did not have the money. They said he will be dead by October 2011, better get things in order.

One morning, as Corrie was trying to get up the stairs, he nearly failed completely. He sat there and in tears realized "My life is over. Time to sail." He knew all his life; he is not going to be a burden in his old day for anybody. When his life time is running out, he will sail off into the sea never to return. This looked like it is that time.

Then in 2011 he retired from the boat factory, leaving it all in the capable hands of his sons. Corrie started to work on the small land he had at that time, farming. By hand, lots of sunshine. Lower stress. He also started on serious diets, it worked in making his lungs a bit better but nothing worked for the weight loss. He underwent treatment by an old Chinese herbalist with cannabis oil, once a day. Sadly that old man passed away and his son is now running the same shop – as a Big Pharma outlet.

Corrie read about the Potato Only diet and during mid-2012 followed that for nearly 4 months. Only potato, nothing else allowed.

He also bought a bicycle, starting off with barely 100 meters a day he worked up to a daily routine of 10 km in the morning. A few weekend trips even pushed it to 50 km over two days. Walking was difficult, but cycling was sort of manageable. That was now if we ignore the painful feeling of weight pushing the small bicycle seat up into places it is not supposed to go. He finally started losing weight. Life got a bit better, though walking and moving around remained extremely painful and difficult. That December 2011 he had to get a medical certificate for his driving license . . .

The hospital got new scales. They could measure up to 250 Kg. There was no more telling the nurse that he is only 162 kg! The scale measured a whopping 187.6 Kg. The only provable record he has. By that time Corrie knew he had already lost a few centimeters in waist line – but this was a real shocker, even for him. Blood pressure was the usual through the roof.

During 2012 and 2013 Corrie tried various diets, worked very hard on the land and pedaled the bicycle for more than 4,500 km in total. It has a speed and odometer on.

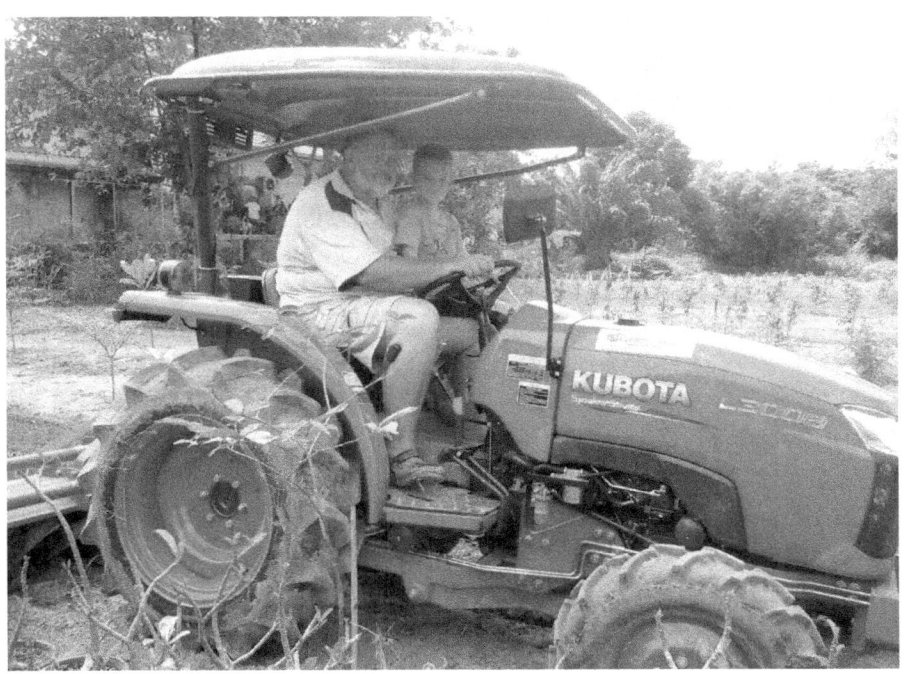

October 2012 – First time I lost a bit of weight in my life.

Finally, at the age of 57 Corrie slowly started losing weight. But – not for long. He got the weight down to 165; but then it relentlessly crawled up again – to 174.7 Kg. From there it would not move lower. Corrie even checked on other scales, same results. 175 Kg it was. That did not even justify new clothes!

For nearly two years that was where he was stuck – 174/175 Kg. To maintain that, he had to remain very strict on diet all the time. But, there was a bright light in the darkness. He slowly gained mobility in his legs and could walk short distances without the crutches, and without too much pain.

Then came the magical day in May 2016. His scale said he lost 2 Kg of weight. Corrie could not believe it. He kept on checking his weight every few hours – the same; he is down by 2 Kg. A week later he was down another 2 Kg, and so the one week fades into the other. By the end of

June 2016, he was down 6 Kg. 8 Kg in July – Excitement filled his fat body right to the bone marrows. He is too scared to say or do anything, just kept every day the same as the previous and trying to figure out what happened. Something is working. Month by month his weight dropped. There is no better motivation for any obese person than seeing the loss of weight, virtually on daily basis. Some months less, some months as much as 12 Kg. Down, down, down. Happy and on to be happier.

Until 4 April 2017 – finally 99.4 Kg. He is now maintaining the weight between 95 and 99 kg. A little problem though, he has to work a bit hard not to lose more weight. He really doesn't want to become skin and bones either.

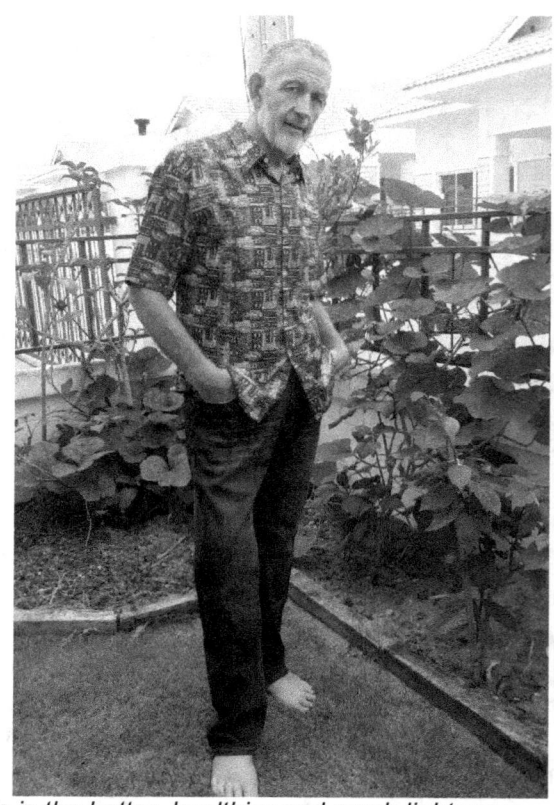

This is the better, healthier and much lighter me.
April 2017.

- Exactly what I did.

Sorry, you suffered all the way until here to learn all I did. Believe me, the rest of this book is important for you to understand — so you can learn to listen to what your body is doing, saying and begging. In this chapter I will describe what I did, how it basically affected me.

However; do make sure to read the more detailed information about the various elements which I am referring to, i.e. Potato Diet, Low Carb High Fat, etc. I did many things, some not a great success, some were plain astonishing. Thus, let me step back to beginning 2014.

I read, studied and watched many videos about the Potato Only diet. I felt I can do it, so I decided to give it a try. Anyway, I love potatoes but it is definitely not going to be possible to eat some 8 Kg per day! So just try and see. A week went by nothing happened. Two weeks and for the first time in my life there was a small drop in weight. The third week I lost 2 Kg – from the start. Wow, I was motivated, I was over excited. I looked more intensely into that Potato diet and I also started cycling. I did lose a LOT of weight, down from the recorded 187.6 kg to just over 165 Kg.

Although I lost that 22 kg in six months, not much was visible, neither did I need to reduce my clothes size. Other people did not even notice any changes.

But then it flat lined. No up, no down. I reduced my potatoes, I increased the cycling, added other exercises. I felt like I can go crazy – my weight did not break down from that 165 Kg. It was my Berlin wall. I started eating normal – but very small portions – and slowly the horror happened. Weight increased, very slowly, very definitely. I got very busy with some other issues, thus weigh control and exercise went a bit out the back door. By March 2016 I was back up to 175 Kg. I started feeling it in my back and legs again.

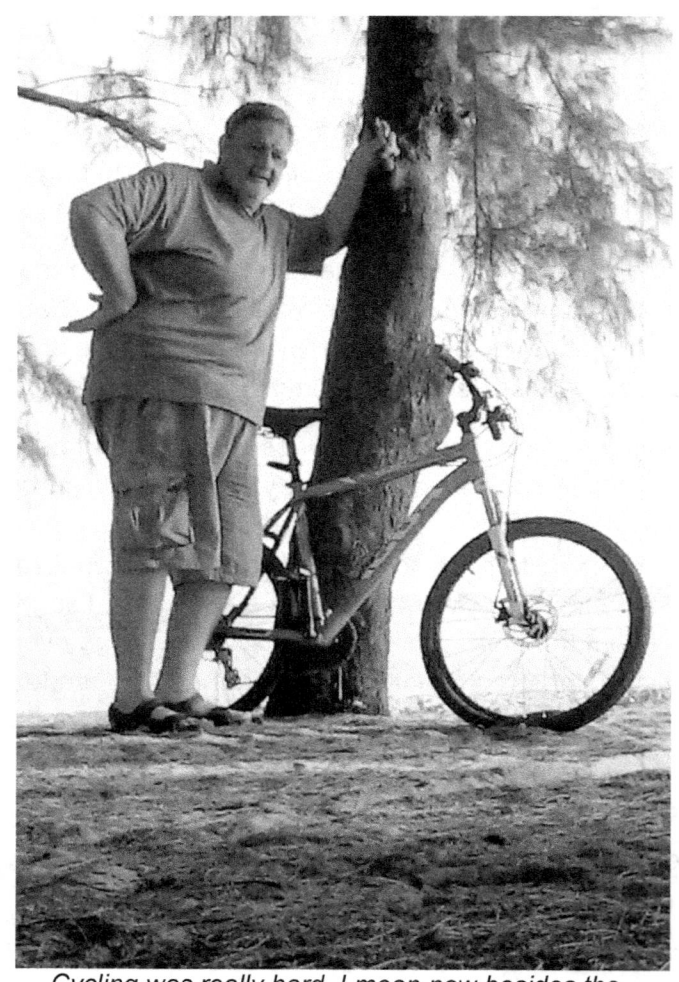

Cycling was really hard, I mean now besides the small thing I had to sit on. But the nice coastal scenery made up for that suffering.

At that time, I learned quite a lot about the alkaline pH hype, many videos, and many documents. Mostly it is about health issues and cancer, but few were able to describe exactly what and why. At that time, I had a big lump on my left forearm, about 8 cm in diameter and about 2 cm thick – still growing. I suspected cancer, maybe a spread from my earlier lung problem; hence my interest in the potential remedies besides cannabis. My Chinese hero sadly passed on to the other side.

I started to drink water throughout the day charged with baking soda. In the morning I dump a heaped teaspoon in a 600 ml bottle of water and finish it through the day time. Also drank other (normal) water in-between. By that time, I was not consuming any other sugars in any form except for the sucrose one get in raw fruits like watermelon and mango. Coffee was still my daily pleasure, but down to one cappuccino in the morning only – wake up time. Nice full cream shop milk and all. And microwaved. Yes, I knew about all the bad stories around microwave ovens, but ignored them in lieu of convenience. And I was still eating three small meals a day and maybe a salad or fruit in evening or afternoon when feeling hungry, which I always did.

A note about microwaves: Is it not funny how so many 'advisors' can tell you that the microwaves is bad for your health. Yet, when asked exactly how it makes out to be bad, they fail to have the logical scientific answer. The same with so many other health issues.

Slowly my weight started to drop again, very slowly. One kg in April and two kg in May. Nothing I can do about that but being happy, it is slowly going down. During those months I started to intensely look into the various weight loss programs, advice, etc.

I discovered the phenomena of 'One Meal A Day' – OMAD. But for me, that was totally stupid and basically impossible. I have problems getting through the day eating three or four small meals, now to even thinking of reducing all of that to only one . . .!

This OMAD thing kept on jumping up in my mind, I found myself time after time getting back to that idea. I tried to get onto that three times in the two months, but I just could not succeed, the hungry suffering was way too much. Rather die a Happy Fat Corrie than suffer like that.

Then I found another concept – Low Carbohydrate, High Fat (LC-HF) diet. That is more acceptable to me than starvation. I like a nice fat strip on the side of my steak, not even to talk about the magical smoked bacon. So I look into that with great interest. The first part – Low Carbohydrate is a bit controversial if you include grains and fiber, but that I could live with. But it was against ALL logic to eat a lot of fatty stuff. What about cholesterol? It was straight up against anything and everything I ever learned about health, diet and weight loss. Luckily, the idea kept stuck in my mind, and I kept coming back to it. I found a number of YouTube videos from people that successfully lost a lot of weight on this concept. But it just did not make sense.

In June 2016 I decided it is time to go for a full weight loss; make or break. I can't keep on living like that. It all happened when I woke at night feeling heavy clamped on my chest. I could feel my heart beating like an African drum, but it missed a few beats on the run. I realized things are probably on the final stage. At least I lived a full five years longer than what they gave me back in 2010.

The next hours and day or two I tried to determine what I can do, considering all I have done in the past. The only issue that did work for me was the Potato Only diet. Thus I went off shopping – Potatoes. (See full chapter on Potato Diet).

For the following 6 weeks I remained strict on the potato diet. After the first week my weight started dropping and I was feeling very happy. Besides that, I was also feeling very good – physically. It is an easy diet in some ways since your stomach does not really feel empty all the time. But you do feel hungry and craving other foods a lot, especially in the beginning.

So what is the reasoning behind this? To fill the stomach and get off the general food concept. For the first few days I maintained three meals a day. After a few days of only potato, it becomes a bit boring. I found myself setting breakfast off for later in the day; around 10h00. Lunch was rather skipped and I enjoyed a nice hour long sleep session more than eating potatoes. By later afternoon I started feeling hollow, time to eat – potatoes. That was usually around 17h00 since I was already long time keeping the law of not eating at least three hours before sleeping time.

The boring potatoes made me also do one thing I did not really do before – the number of potatoes that I could eat reduced. From somewhere around four or five potatoes (1 Kg) down to about one (250 gram) per meal.

Then one day I was entrenched in the story I was writing, after breakfast. I did not realize the time until darkness. About 19h30 I realized I am not really feeling hungry and definitely do not feel like cooking potato. I went to sleep. The next morning, I woke up – still no hungry feeling. I monitored myself very carefully and tried that for a few days. I ate 2 potatoes in the morning and every other day nothing in the evening. I felt really very good. Including very energetic.

I realized the "One Meal A Day" concept was within my reach, maybe for a few days at a time.

June and July I lost about 6 Kg each of the two months.

So what happened?

My body was adopting to the potato as sole food source. More important that that; the Hunger Hormones did not wake up anymore, especially the Insulin production remained on a bottom flat line. Because the insulin dropped, other hormones could extract the stored fat from the cells to maintain the energy in the body. It did not last very long.

Beginning of August my weight drop stopped again. For a bit more than ten days I did not lose even 100 grams; yet I was still on the same diet. I also started feeling tired, needed more sleep. By that time, I was fully on a One Meal a Day program.

Then I changed my step and went for the High Fat diet. Ever since, until now I am on this system. It is quite fun to cook for myself, it is a diet loaded with energy and good feeling and good tasty eating.

16 September 2016 I stood on 147.2 Kg – the first photo record.

I found that my stomach definitely shrank, I could not eat more potatoes than the one or sometimes two tubers. Here is where listening to your body comes in too. Sometimes your body say "Stop the fat, I need a rest." Ok fine, stop eating any fatty foods. Those days I usually find myself a bit lazy (low energy) and the easiest thing to cook is . . . potato.

12 October 2016 – down to 139.8 Kg. A very happy day, another boundary crossed.

ALWAYS remember – if you eat potato, then do not, NEVER, eat any other kinds of food at least six hours before and six hours after. Thus, I will cook potato and that will be all I eat for the whole day, or two. Drink only water. It is amazing how your energy goes up and your physical feelings are happy.

My weight kept on dropping. On my birthday, fourth of December 2016, I reached my original dream target for the year; to be below 130 Kg. I was a wonderful 127.4 Kg. I never thought that would ever be possible again, but there it was.

Sometimes it slows down, maybe 1 Kg in two weeks. It was in November that I realized there is a trigger in my body. In my case, it is set off by watermelon. Yes, quite a funny thing to realize, and I proved it to myself by causing a few 'trigger events'. Some days while on the High Fat – with only One Meal A day in the morning – I feel a bit underfed by late afternoon. Then I will eat some fruits, mostly fatty like Avocado or the sweetness of a watermelon slice. Just a cup full. Usually the next day weight is reducing again. Is it because of the diuretic effect from watermelon or is it something else? I will give the answer in the chapter about Watermelon.

On the 4th of February 2017 I broke through the last targeted barrier of 110 Kg. My magical dream weight of 109.6 kg. I made myself a serious promise – "I will not go through 110 Kg upwards again. Even if it means I stop eating 100%.

Although that was what I dreamed, my absolute wish for this past few decades; I find that I still have a bit of belly fat. That needs to go away, so I decided to slow down on the speed of weight loss, but still let it go on until my tummy skin is less than 15 mm when folded.

There you have it, all of this book about this short story. But, you need to understand what is happening, you need to have a good idea of why it is happening. The rest of this book I will expand on the background information.

Now, on 4 April 2017 – 10 months since I seriously started with this adventure; I am down to 98 Kg.

Maybe you will wonder what it feels like to be half your old size. So let me just spend a little to tell you about this magic feeling. Let us call it "Motivation".

- The New Life.

I don't think I need to expand much about the life I had as Big Corrie. The suffering starts in the night, sleep is not long. I needed to go to the toilet with full bladder about every two or three hours. Now to do such a thing was quite an effort. First I have to get my head up from the pillow, swing my legs off the bed and sit there for a minute or two. Just to get the blood back into my brain and to 'wake my legs up'. Then I will pull myself up against the wardrobe and stand there for another minute or two before I can dare to take a step. Getting to the toilet had its own difficulties. Getting back on bed was relative easy. Rolling over on my bed (only a single wide bed) was also an effort, could not do that in my sleep. I had to shuffle this way, push that way. If I would roll from my left side to my right side; I would be on the floor before the half turn.

Then comes the day. Breakfast, lunch and dinner. Hungry in between, coffee time in the morning, tea time in the late noon. All the time I promised myself "Tomorrow I will start my dieting again". Tomorrow never comes.

Going to visit people had its own problems. Usually they do not have big enough comfortable chairs for Big Corrie; especially at the dinner table. Sitting on a normal chair often came to a crashing disaster of broken chairs. Oh, yea I had quite a number of those under me. There is this one restaurant with fabulous food in Koh Kong, Cambodia. Just over the border from Thailand, some 7 km. 'Fat Sam' had special chairs there for people like Sam and me. Big, comfortable and very sturdy, made from bamboo. When big people walks in there, the staff is quickly to guide you to one of the three Special Chairs. I am still looking forward to visit them again, soon. Can only imagine the faces when they see me. I should give a free copy of this book to Sam. Sam is an amazing personality, always ready to help wherever he can, stunning memory for people's names.

What a nightmare to go somewhere in any form of public transport, including aircrafts. I am a bit on the tall side, so in itself already a problem in Asian transports. But then adding a lot of width to the equation makes life for me and neighboring fellow travelers very difficult. The on-board toilet was an absolute impossible option. Just the thought of a long flight where I needed to use the toilet . . . well, I did not take a long flight for more than 8 years.

Let me not expand on the problems at some bus doors or walking down the narrow alley to your seat. Hence I only used that option when there is really no other. Sitting on a chair the first problem is my knees, they are hard pressed against the chair in front of me. Second off course are the armrests, if they can't lift up, I can't sit there. After the first half an hour it is difficult to rate which is the worst; knee pain, cramping legs, back pain, shoulder pain ... or the facial expressions of whomever is punished to sit next to me.

Buying clothes. I have been living in Pattaya for about 12 years now. For the most of this time, the only place I could get my size 66 pants or 6XL shirt like tents were in a shop in Bangkok. The only other option was to have things tailor made – expensive. Thus, if I needed a new T-Shirt it required me the trip to MBK center in Bangkok, 180 km there and 180 km back – with horrible traffic all the way. For the last few years there is a tourist trap in Pattaya that started selling these Super-Size clothes, so that made the issue a bit better.

Besides all the drama of getting things, they are also much more expensive. Oh, and do not forget the additional weight. My carry-on bag for flights could take one jean, 2 T-shirts, 1 sleeve shirt, one short and maybe a small towel; then I am over the 7 Kg allowance. Now I can easily take two jeans, a long trouser, two shorts and 4 shirts with towel and extras.

I can walk into most shops and they have my new size 40 pants and the lose LL shirts are plentiful.

On the issue of flights. I started hearing this motion that some airliners are going to charge a penalty rate for people that are so far over weight. Like paying extra for the extra kilograms on the passenger. I did fear those days because I think I will explode in anger. Will they give discounts for small underweight people? Well, somehow I can understand it too. Now, it would not matter to me anymore.

Driving a car: I did not really notice how much space there are in even small cars, ever. Until my weight dropped to under the 120 kg mark. Amazing how far the steering wheel is now, I have to stretch. Somewhat of a mystery, why am I sitting so low in the seat?

Lately I was not really driving much anywhere. Thus it was the first time in January 2017 that I suddenly noticed all the changes in my seven-year-old Isuzu. Lots of cabin space, the steering wheel is now at least 25 cm from my tummy, there is a great increase in the space between my head and roof. I am literally sitting lower in the car. On closer inspection I found the reasons, and estimates. I sit at least 7 cm lower – because my big ass is no more. I sit at least 6 cm further back, because the thick layer of fat on my back is no more present. My arms are right next to my body, comfortable; because there are no more pillows under my armpits. To try explain the exact feeling I will need to go back many years in my life. Sitting in my what-used-to-be-normal Isuzu truck was OK, best for my size anyway. But now I feel like a ten-year-old kid getting illegally behind the steering wheel of his dad's car! The car has gone so BIG. Or is it me that shrunk?

Things are not always only good. I do not have my build in cushions anymore. Sitting on a hard surface is damn uncomfortable, sometimes really painful on my poor coccyx bones. The bones of my spine and shoulders are now only covered by skin, no more soft padding. Thus sitting with my back against a hard surface is . . . well it is hard. Even my shoes are a bit big, because of the narrowness of my feet and much less fat on the bridge of my feet. Hey, there are small spaces between my toes, never before in my life!

Walking is awkward, I find myself leaning forward. That is because I do not have the big weight in front to pull me forward anymore. Now I still need to find a new balance in my body.

Then there is this one very strange thing. I truly do not know my own body, not at all. I don't even know myself anymore. Looking in a glass reflection and even a mirror is still a shock. I see this stranger looking back at me, thin, looks older, just looks so very strange. Walking (gait) has changed.

But the worst is the new 'feeling' when touching my own strange body. Washing my back and shoulders, I am still riddled to this day to feel the bones. Bumping the front of my leg against something is a hell of lot more painful, only bone and skin.

One day about two months ago I was still relaxing on bed after waking in the morning. Felt a little pain on my lower abdominal side. Rubbing there with my hand, I had a sudden rude awakening. There is one hell of a lump where it is not supposed to be. I was immediately very alarmed – What now? Cancer growth is the thing that jumped to my mind. Upon further careful investigation, I found it is my hip bone and it hurt because a small pillow was under it for some time during sleeping. I never realized how much the bones were hidden by thick layers of fat in my previous body.

Itching on my cheek. Another very strange feeling to have skin and bone there – not the soft fat padding that I had all my life. Under my chin, around my neck was a permanent sleeping pillow, now that is gone. Fortunately, there the skin is not too loose after the size reduction. But the strange thing – and believe me, this was another bit of a stare on my part. I could see my Adams-apple; first time in my whole life I can see that knob.

Well, that is the new me. I will have to get used to it. But I tell you this; it is a great pleasure to get up from sleeping, straight up, no pause and immediately walk to toilet. It is wonderful not to worry about the survivability of the chair you are going to sit on. Getting on public transport is a hell of a lot more comfortable and cheaper. I can also consider buying a smaller car next time. Smaller and cheaper clothes.

Where before I needed all the muscular power in my arms to lift my massive body out of a chair; now I usually stand up without even using my arms to press on anything. Just lean forward and get up on my legs.

You know for instance; I have a small 7 Kg washing machine. Only two set of clothes and it was full. Now I put four sets of clothes plus a towel or two and there is space for more.

Then there is the Big Bonus. Although I did not push very strongly for this, the whole system of weight loss had an extra spin off. My blood pressure is now on a normal 'healthy' average 138/82/64 (Down from the extreme danger 185/120/65).

Oh yes. One last thing I noticed only a month or so ago: My lower legs were severely covered with ugly varicose veins. Both my father and mother went in their early 50's to have them surgically tugged, thus I know . . . Now, astonishingly, it is nearly cleared off. Only on my right calf is a small patch of maybe 10 sq/cm remaining, and not so bulging heavy – still fading visibly every week.

- My personal daily routine.

Nothing is set in stone, I change often. To get into a very rigid routine is boring. Yes, it is good (maybe very good) for you to develop an extreme kind of routine. Maybe Aerobics or hard sweating in the gym. I am not yet on that level. Currently I am still working on balance and mobility. Due to being extreme obese, I did spend years not moving much. The results are that all my joints were basically limited in their movement, by tendons and bone growth. My spine used to be rigid and near inflexible. Thus I started off with walking, swinging arms and twisting spine. Now that I am more flexible and joints are loose; I can work on building muscle again.

The following is my basic daily routine, probably 80% of the time. Sometimes more activities added, sometimes more time on the writing – or a few times the whole routine is scrapped because I go out etc.

I usually wake up around 05h00 in the morning. That is the best time for me to start writing. First thing I do, while on the bed, is to do my series of breathing exercises. Then I make a cup of herbal tea. Yes, tea – no coffee anymore. Most of the time it is freshly cut ginger and cinnamon. This I drink while checking Facebook and other sites of news and interesting things. Spend about 30 minutes, slowly sipping on the hot tea. I can feel it landing in my much smaller stomach and soothing all over the body. Then I review whatever I wrote the previous days; that is now with relation to articles and book writing.

Around 07h00 in the morning I start my exercise routines, walking my rubbish to the bins and a few extra lengths gives me a relaxing 1.2 km. Sometimes I walk this two or three times. Back at home I do my stretching, swinging and twisting exercises and a few routines with one or two small 5 Kg hand weight. In total I have 24 routines and it takes 55 minutes. When I started off I could barely do 3 or 5 of a routine in total, now I push it to 100 cycles in two minutes.

Finishing that, around 08h30; I will drink some freshly squeezed lemon juice (For Vitamin-C and stomach balancing), then work in my garden for an hour or two. All this with only a short because part of this routine is to expose as much skin to the sun as possible for Vitamin-D. Off course, if there is no sun, or raining then the garden session is out and I do the exercises inside my house. This then followed by a shower and relaxing flat on the floor a bit.

This is the time I check my weight, after morning routine and shower – before eating anything. Currently I am also working on my blood pressure, so Monday, Wednesday and Friday is checking blood pressure, three times each day to get the average.

I will prepare my 'breakfast' which is my main and only big meal a day. Eating about 10h00. Eat slowly and enjoy. Because this is the only 'big' meal I will have all day, I take care to ensure it is tasty, nice, enjoyable and above all – highly nutritious with vitamins and minerals. Then I will do whatever is on the agenda until 12h00. I will take a very enjoyable lunchtime cat-nap rest for up to an hour.

From 13h00 until about 20h00 I am sitting at the computer, writing or doing research. All this time I try to drink as much water as possible. If I feel very hollow (sort of hungry) I will eat something light and small around 16h00 in the afternoon. This might be some fruit, vegetable salad or soup.

All through the day I am trying to maintain at least 1.5 liters of iced water, sometimes herbal tea with honey. In the evening I go shower, relax on bed with YouTube video until I sleep. I usually sleep from 21h00 until 05h00 next day – mobile phone off.

This is the basic, which I try to maintain. Logically it is not always possible since I may get visitors, or need to go shopping, or this or that. Sometimes I write from waking up until maybe 10h00 – then I start the rest of my routines, especially when I feel the need for more sunshine. However, the one rule that stand quite fixed: Main meal somewhere between 10h00 and 11h00 – even if travelling. Maybe a light meal – very light - around 4 pm. Drink lots of water only. No other eat at any other time.

Sleep at least 7 hours at night and try an additional hour around midday.

Get at least 30 minutes of sunshine on as much as possible skin every possible day – and this is very important.

Some sunshine is a lot healthier than no sunshine on your skin. Do not fear the big Pharma hype about all the problems …

I'm getting a little sick and tired of all the little stories your scientists tell about me. Been giving Earth everything it needs for millions of years and now you humans insist **I'M THE PROBLEM??** I'm not impressed!

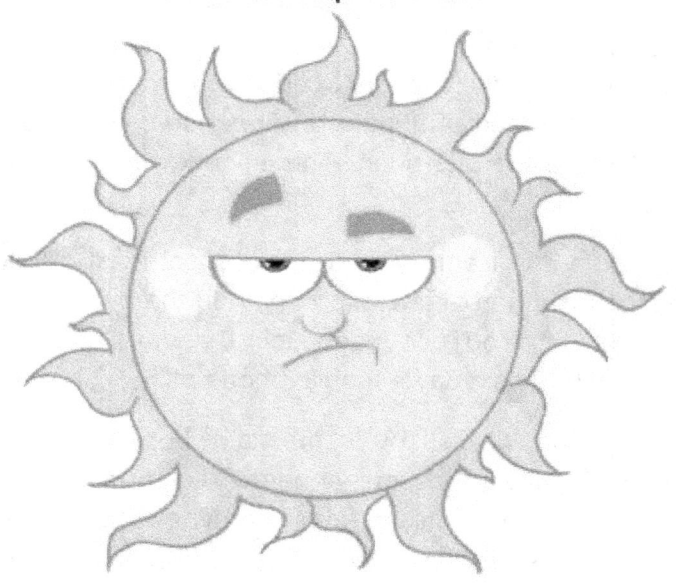

Chapter 2 - Weight Loss.

- Where you will lose weight.

Men and woman lose weight differently and they gain different too. This is a general phenomenon but it might not always be the full story.

Men (usually) lose weight on their body in the following order: Legs, arms, shoulders, chest, back and last of all where we really want to lose weight – stomach.

Women on the other hand lose first on their breasts, then their tummy, fore arms, back and last where they usually wish it was first – legs, hips and upper arms.

The one who pointed this to me many years ago had quite an interesting story behind it. The men need to hunt for food, thus their legs are more important for higher speed. The reason why the tummy is the last to go – that is their reserves during the hunting when they might need to go a few days without food.

Women on the other hand – their bodies protect the womb at all cost. They lose on the breast to tell the men they need to go hunting. Losing weight on the lower body is to make the womb more comfortable. Women is not supposed to be the hunters, therefore their legs and upper arms are rather used as their food storage.

I wonder what will happen now that all of the food gathering, house holding, cooking and baby feeding are changing. Will be interesting to see how the humans re-develop.

How about Body Shape?

Basically there are three types of obese people, each with its own series of problems and challenges. Mostly, the shape of the body can indicate where the problem lies. By no means is this scientifically proven, it is based on a few amateur researchers but no peer reviews

I could find. Personally, I think there are a good amount of merits. Look into this for yourself and see.

Type 1: All body in excess.

This person is obese, from head to toe. The torso, the hips, the legs, arms, neck – everywhere. I was in this category. Now the reason why I post these descriptions is to maybe help you select which way to go with your diet program; especially the pH controls.

This person usually has an effective digestive system and pancreas. There is plenty of insulin in the body, thus easy storage of nutrients in the cell. To be effective in the digestive system, it means a good function from mouth, through stomach, intestines, colon, liver, spleen and pancreas. This person's body is able to extract most nutrients from the food . . . and store that which is in surplus.

It is extremely difficult for this person to lose weight. A sluggish Thyroid gland is often the main culprit for this person; especially low levels of iodine. Increase the consumption of minerals is of critically importance to this person.

The weight loss program for this person would be to reduce the insulin levels in his blood. He would also benefit greatly by increasing the pH of the stomach. Main target for the potato diet would be to change the eating habits and volume. The best and most effective system will be the Low Carbohydrate, High Fat diet – for the rest of his life.

Type 2: Big tummy.

A very common problem with men when they get older. The legs, hips, arms, neck and chest remains relatively good shape. But the tummy is excessive. In general this person can easily lose a few kg of weight with diet; bit not lose a lot and usually does not keep the weight down.

This person most likely has a deficiency in the digestive system, probably the stomach acid and most likely the liver. If you notice the symptoms of mineral deficiency on the nails (especially toe nails) hair and a bit more hidden; rheumatism in the joints; then go to the stomach. It is most likely due to low acidity, high pH. This person needs to increase the stomach acid, which in turn will increase break down of minerals and fix the body.

Often this person will have a mineral deficiency. A good starting point is to increase minerals by supplements.

If this person is somewhat craving for a bit more fatty foods; and if there are no other symptoms on the skin, nails or joints; then this person will have to look at the liver. They might find a problem to digest certain fatty foods, they might regularly experience constipation.

Type 3: Big hips and bums.

This is more typically a gender hormone problem. It is also predominantly a female issue, not many men develop this body shape. Here the main culprit is hormones, in particular oestrogen (estrogen) in women and testosterone in men.

Currently it seems these hormones has a normal controlling effect on the brain. As we get older, their production and presence in our bodies are reducing. That then causes and failure in the brain; somehow reflecting to fat storage around the lower torso; hips, tummy and bums.

This is the only over weight problem where genetics are probably playing a major role.

I did not do much research on this section of the Obese Family, yet.

Keep an eye on my Facebook page and website for more updates.

- Understanding Your Digestive System.

Obviously I can't go into a whole Anatomy and Physiology course here. Just for the sake of interest, the first time I learned about the workings of our own bodies was when I started learning about Alternative Medicine in 1982. Later I did a full qualification as Grade Two Nurse, including a bit more than 1,200 hours of ER hospital duties. Also did a few emergency (First Responder) courses and finally in early 1990's I had to do the whole two-year Anatomy and Physiology course again to qualify for my Aromatherapy Certification. Besides this, I have always been checking in on newer developments and discoveries in the medical field and our own bodies. Quite interesting to know how many issues I was taught and had to write exams on some 35 years ago – now so many are proven wrong! The mainstream medical science is slowly catching up with the alternative.

One particular field of health that has experienced a near complete U-turn is the all-time cursed word DIET. You will find in the later chapters just how far things are upside down with the normal understanding still stuck in people's mind.

When I first learned about the body, one particular disease was always of great interest to me. CANCER. Especially stomach cancer. My father lost half of his life after he was diagnosed with stomach cancer and had a large portion of his stomach and duodenum removed. In 1985, after lots of suffering he died at age of 57 years. So, when I studied this issue, it was generally believed that such cancer were the results of smoking and stress. How wrong they were!

Ever since 1982 there came a new culprit on the horizon; though the majority of medical professionals refused to accept it. Today the picture is so different. The biggest single cause of cancer in the stomach, lower esophagus and duodenum is caused by a little bacteria called 'Helicobacter pylori (H. pylori)'. That is now a proven, all accepted fact. Well, in most cases; however, some still believe the older reasons.

Interesting enough, the second most cause for digestive related cancers is another microbe; *Candida Albicans*.

Why I mention this – *H. Pylori* is something you need to know about and watch out for IF you want to do what I did in losing so much weight. More about these two big problems later. For now, let us just get back to the digestive system and how it operates – in relation to our weight loss quest.

We eat food, through our mouth into the stomach, then after just a few minutes (or hours) it passes to the duodenum and eventually into the small intestines from where the blood absorbs that which it needs. Whatever remains goes to the colon and out the back hole all of us are equipped with. That is the short version, but we need to take a more in depth look at this.

We eat …

Why do we eat?

Because we are hungry or because we like the taste? Or just because it is time to eat? Where did this concept of three meals a day came from, with coffee break and tea break and night snack all in between? It might come as a massive surprise to most people. Your body only need you to eat one time a day. In short it is often called OMAD – 'One Meal A Day'.

When we are born, we need to eat many times a day; around ten times. Then as toddler it will change down to four times, as teenager, when we are on that 'fast stretch time' we will eat just about all day. Around the twenty years of age, we are done growing and the demand for food from the body reduces. Maybe still on a three meal a day, though it is where the problem usually starts. By the time we pass thirty years of age, the slowing metabolism does not need to eat more than twice a day. By the age of forty – one good meal a day is more than sufficient.

The moment you bring food towards your mouth, your body is already preparing to digest that. As you chew, the food is being processed and mixed with enzymes in your saliva. Even before the food reaches to your stomach, just the smell and taste of it in your mouth sets of a long range of notifications and alarm bells through your body. Your stomach is preparing to receive the food by releasing hydrochloric acid. Your pancreas is manufacturing insulin and other hormones, your liver is making bile and other chemicals, pumping it to the gall bladder. Amazing, all that before you swallow the first bite. Now you swallow the food, it moves down the esophagus, pass through a very critical valve into the stomach.

In the stomach the food is mixed with hydrochloric acid. The acidity (pH) in a normal healthy stomach is between 1.5 and 3.5 – very acidic. Being of Hydrochloric acid; if you take that stomach content out and pour it on iron, it will even corrode the iron; just like the industrial acid you can buy or which some people use in their swimming pools. Remember this if you one day may need to break out from a prison!

Your stomach is a very special organ; it is made in such way that it can withstand this extreme acid. At the inlet to your stomach there is a valve, the *lower esophagus valve*. This valve has two functions, to prevent unwanted material entry to the stomach i.e. food which your taste buds already determined as not suitable and often also food to which your body has a natural intolerance. The other, much more important purpose, is to prevent the strong hydrochloric acid (HCL) from getting into your *esophagus* since that will cause problems.

Again, this is where we learned something wrong. A major mistake on which the big Pharmaceutical companies makes billions of dollars without helping you right. See, that Acid-reflux and/or Heartburn of which we so suffer … You know the one where you grab a Rennie, Eno, baking soda, alkaline water or some other anti-acid and get such magical quick relief?

The whole understanding is actually wrong. You do not suffer from too much acid in your stomach – you actually have too little stomach acid! If your stomach is more alkaline (pH higher than 3.5); you will not really feel any discomfort. THAT is until and unless or when the still acidic liquid in your stomach starts pushing up past the *lower esophagus valve.* The burning sensation you feel – it is acid coming into your food downpipe; which is not made to handle such acidic substances.

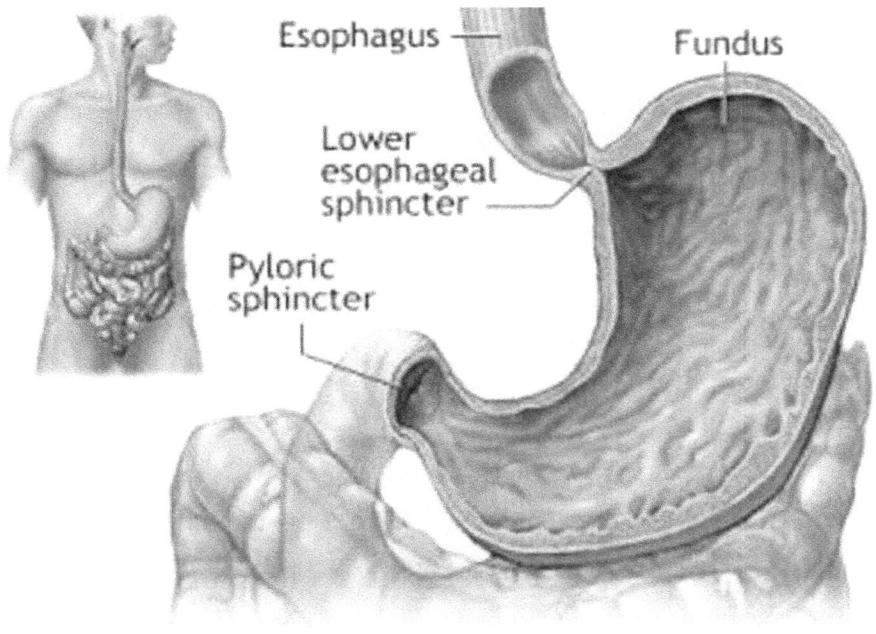

Diagram showing the stomach with inlet and outlet sphincters.

- CRITICAL INFO:

The *lower esophagus valve* operates with acid, no conscious or unconscious control from the brain at all. IF and while the pH (acid level) in your stomach is between 1.5 and 3.5 (or lower); this valve will remain closed; in such way that it acts as a one-way control. Food stuff can only go down into the stomach. As soon as anything acidic comes in contact with this valve, from the stomach side, it will clamp shut.

Thus, when your stomach pH level is say 4.0; then this valve may remain relaxed to acidic fluids from the stomach, and such may push up into your food pipe, the esophagus. That will cause discomfort.

That of course is provided you do not have a physical failure or damage to this valve!

On the outlet side of your stomach, leading to the duodenum there is another valve; the *pyloric sphincter*. This valve is exactly the opposite of the inlet to the stomach. Its main function is to control the flow of whatever pass through to the duodenum and small intestines. It is a security guard, major safety mechanism. Water has a near free pass to go through, some other material also. But anything fatty, minerals or any form of protein does not pass unless it is well mixed and dissolved by the HCL and enzymes in your stomach. Not acidic enough, not dissolved; no pass. Full stop.

Thus, in short, the inlet valve prevents acid stuff from going back up to your throat while the outlet valve only allows digested stuff to pass into the rest of your body.

There is one other point I will need to explain here. The much hated, little known, mostly ignored little bug that most of us has in our stomach. The fearsome *H. Pylori*. This nasty screw like bug can be there in your stomach fighting the acidic environment for many years, even as long as 70 years. Normally it does not harm you, it does not bother your body. It is just there, surviving in your gut and trying to make the environment more acceptable for its own species to explode in many little babies.

See, this thing can only survive in an alkaline environment. However, it has a mucus type of secretion that it can cover itself with and that allows it to remain even in the harshness of your stomach walls. All the time, this little gogga is trying to reduce the acidity of its environment. It wants to make your stomach more alkaline.

Since part of this procedure I did was making my stomach less acidic, it fits right into the wishes of this *H. Pylori*; and they exploded. Yip, due to lack of knowledge around January 2017 the *H. Pylori* population exploded. But I learned, I coped and eventually I conquered.

Hence; you will benefit from this book more than you can imagine. See later chapter about *Conquer H. Pylori.* This is a VERY critically operation to understand.

Next the food will pass through the duodenum where the HCL acidity is neutralized with bile from the liver and many different substances are added to the biomass to mark various nutrients and make them all absorbable by the blood throughout the small intestines. The passage of the food through the approximately six meters intestine takes between three and six hours.

Finally, it is queued up in the colon, some nutrient and mostly water is absorbed from here while most of the waste material from the body is also added here. The food remains a staggering 20 to 40 hours in your colon. If your system is fast acting good peristalsis and very healthy the total time from eat to disposal should be around 24-hours. Some constipation, not good balance in food, too much solids then it can take even as long as 60-hours.

Now, this is not the law, not even of averages. It will depend very much on what you consume. Water passes through in minutes, juices like from a slight acidic smoothie can take 15-minutes. A heavy steak meal can take 5-hours; a spicy chili meal takes two hours. Funny enough cow or goat milk takes about two hours while white steamed fish will pass through in about 30-minutes.

Thus what does that mean for our eating habits? It means what you eat can make you feel full for a longer or shorter period of time. On the overall, if you eat heavy things that stays for longer time in your body, it also means the digestive system is slowing down. Becoming congested. So when you force the next meal in while the previous one is not yet done ... guess what happens. Your body needs to make a plan, so much energy just lying there. Your body starts to absorb more nutrients than what it needs and deposits it in cells for storage. The last thing you want is to store lots of food in your cells. It is stored as fat and it makes you fat.

But let us take one step back in this process. Why do we eat? Normally the answer is because we are hungry. However, most often the feeling of 'hungry' should rather be 'craving'. Especially with us overweight people, we eat because we crave something. "If I can only lose my appetite." Or "If I can just stop wanting that morning coffee."

Well, I took a long hard look at this single concept. I think this is the most critically important thing for you to understand.

- Why do we feel hungry?

Surprise – you do not feel hungry because your stomach is empty and now cramping from hunger! In fact, there is very little sensory nerve communication between your stomach and the brain – and the brain is the part which tells you what is happening in your body.

The communication with regards to hunger feeling – or rather 'want to eat' is by means of hormones. These hormones are excreted into the bloodstream and swirl around there until it reaches the sensory glands in your brain. If we can somehow prevent these from reaching the brain, we can probably lose weight more easily. Indeed, but would it not be better to prevent the excess of these hormones to even be manufactured and released in the first place?

Well, that is where we are going to start.

- The Hungry Hormones.

Ahh, there you are, you silly rascal. Let's eliminate them, get it out of my body!

Oops, sorry you cannot.

Without this most active hormone you will not live to see the end of this day.

In fact, (to current knowledge) there are three hormones that controls your 'feeling hungry'. Two of them still relatively little studied. But there is one that is very dominant, and in our whole existence that one is the most important one.

The lesser two hormones are called Ghrelin and Leptin. Almost sounds like the monsters of Gremlins. Ghrelin makes you feel hungry, increase appetite. Leptin is just the opposite; causes you to feel full and reduces appetite. If your diet is in balance and you are receiving adequate SLEEP, they perform in perfect symphony. However, if your diet is in chaos and your sleep is little, they go haywire. The funny thing with these two is that they are most affected by the micronutrients that you consume, rather than how much you eat. Know the feeling of being hungry after you just ate a big BBQ? Yip that is Ghrelin telling you it still fails to find the micronutrients your body seeks.

Besides the micronutrients, there is one more way to control these two rascals. Get enough sleep! Yip, if you sleep more, the Ghrelin goes to sleep too. Guess what? You do not feel so hungry anymore. Or, maybe it is your body that is able enough to transmute (Manufacture) many of the nutrients it requires while you sleep.

The University of Chicago conducted a study in 2004 and again in 2013 to see if sleep deprivation altered appetite. They tested men who slept 4 hours for two consecutive nights followed by 10 hours of sleep for two consecutive nights. They found that after sleeping for 4 hours versus the 10, the men had an average 18% lower levels of Leptin (Make you feel not hungry) and an average 28% higher Ghrelin levels (the one that makes you hungry) during the short sleep days. During the short sleep days, the subject stated they feel much hungrier than usual and craved salty, sweet food. In summary, sleep deprivation not only increases hunger levels, but lowers metabolism, not a good combination for health and weight loss.

Now, this next is the BIG hormone. The boss of it all. Do you know that most overweight people also has at least a bit of diabetic problems? Think diabetes, think insulin.

- The Insulin as Hunger Hormone.

Insulin is made in the pancreas and allows cells to absorb sugars from the blood stream and convert them to energy. In the western world insulin problems are most likely one of the major causes of the majority of diseases. From bacterial infections, virus attacks, headaches right on to Cancer and other serious diseases like Alzheimer's, dementia, etc.

Approximately one-third of the population has a resistance to respond properly to insulin, which prompts the pancreas to secrete more insulin if you eat a meal high in refined or "simple" carbohydrates such as refined sugar, white pasta or white bread.

When the insulin does not respond normally, you can experience insulin induced hunger; or should we rather say it correct - a gnawing desire to eat. If you consume meals high in refined carbohydrates on a regular basis you will continually crave more carbohydrates, the more your pancreas release insulin to digest, the more you crave . . . a vicious cycle. The more refined carbohydrates you consume, the more your energy levels fluctuate between high and low throughout the day.

If you have other mineral and vitamin problems in your body and the most critical is a pH error, then insulin just cannot do its normal work. Then insulin sends emergency alarms to the brain for more food; you eat more, the balance gets worse, more alarms, more eat . . .

Typically, like any factory worker, your body is lazy. It prefers to have lots of carbohydrates or sugars to use as energy fuel rather than anything else. And stored fats in the body is the most difficult to convert back to use as fuel. Your body may not tap into your fat stores if you are trying to lose weight. If you continue on a diet with sugar and simple carbohydrates, your body will prompt you to continue eating these foods, leading to increased hunger and chronic carbohydrate cravings.

The positive tradeoff that you will experience is that when your body start using the stored fat, you will have more energy. One gram of fat has a lot more energy than one gram of sugar.

CRITICAL POINT:

While you have high insulin in your blood, the body can't withdraw stored energy (read body fat) from the cells to utilize. I repeat; "If your insulin levels are high, you cannot lose weight"! Full stop. Rather, the opposite happens. Insulin forces more nutrients into the cells, cells expand – and you gain weight.

So here my dear friends are one of the very critical points to understand in this whole program. Do not cause a spike in your insulin production by the pancreas. If you can keep this, and you can reduce the requirements of insulin by the body – THEN the minerals like Magnesium and other hormones can begin to withdraw fat from the cells and convert it to energy.

Then you WILL lose weight.

- The Other Hormone – Cortisol.

Although Cortisol is not a 'hungry feeling' hormone – it is an important hormone in the weight loss program. The main problem with Cortisol is that it prevents the re-absorption of fat from the body cells. Cortisol is secreted by the adrenal kidneys. For any weight loss program, Cortisol is a very big problem; and it is a direct stress related hormone.

For losing weight we do need to reduce the secretion of Cortisol. One of the main methods is to reduce stress, better to eliminate all forms of stress completely. A good way to reduce stress is walking, not really big exercise. Increase the potassium intake and Vitamin B1, preferably a natural or yeast supplement like Marmite or Vegemite. The next reducer is sleep. You have to sleep more than 8 hours per day. Add into this mix is Sunshine, which will enable the body to manufacture Vitamins D, especially D3. If you can't get at least 30 minutes sunshine per day, then you will need to use supplements.

Personally, I like to get around one hour of sunlight per day, working in the garden or just relaxing on the lawn; somewhere between 09h00 and 12h00 on the day or in late afternoon. The sun here in Pattaya (Thailand) is very strong.

- Insulin, Sugar and Fat.

Just to get your mind in a good spin, I am going to jump in with a quote from the book "Textbook of Medical Physiology" by Guyton and Hall; page 930.

"When the GLUCOSE concentration is low, INSULIN secretion by the pancreas is suppressed and FAT is utilized almost exclusively for energy everywhere except in the brain; when the glucose concentration is high, insulin secretion is stimulated, and carbohydrate is utilized instead of fat until the excess blood glucose is stored in the form of liver glycogen or muscle glycogen. Therefore, one of the most important functional roles of insulin in the body is to control which of these two foods, from moment to moment, will be used by the body for energy."

Insulin increases the absorption of glucose into the cells, muscles and liver. It converts sugars into stored glycogen, cholesterol, triglycerides and fat. In effect it prevents fat from being used.

This is a very important fact to understand. If you do not have high levels of insulin – then your body will be able to use stored fats from the cells to burn as energy. You need to reduce the insulin levels the natural way; by not eating any foods that are insulin demanding. No carbohydrates, etc. There is also another issue here. Every time you eat anything; the moment food lands in your stomach, the pancreas starts pumping insulin. Thus the next step, after cutting insulin demanding foods, is eat less times. Intermittent fasting is the right way.

The opposing force of insulin is the 'Hormone Sensitive Lipase - HSL'. The main function of hormone-sensitive lipase is to mobilize the stored fats. HSL is activated when the body needs to mobilize energy stores. It frees cholesterol back to be used as stored energy. It is inhibited by insulin. The higher the insulin, the lower the HSL and the less fat can be withdrawn to be used for energy - and more sugars are stored as fat.

Carbohydrates initially lowered the appetite, but then rebounded soon afterward with a vengeance causing the appetite to be even greater than before the food was introduced. Eating carbohydrates in combination with any other foods, makes the other go into storage as fat.

Let us look at some concepts on how to reduce your insulin spikes. Normally you should eat some protein in your main meal; daily. Protein does somewhat suppress the appetite, especially insulin triggered.

Together with proteins comes fats. Be it from fruits like avocado or a nice piece of steak, various kinds of nuts, butter grilled pumpkin; it does not matter. Fat has a neutral effect on appetite; and no effect on insulin.

Nutrients can only be stored in the cells of the body while insulin is present in the blood. Thus if you do not have lots of insulin escorting the nutrients; they cannot enter into the cells – they cannot be stored and you cannot get fat.

- The body pH – Acidity or Alkalinity.

Oh my world, is there a controversy about this topic.

If there is one part in this book that you truly need to understand and study very well, it is this chapter about the pH. This is where you can make or break your health, where you can learn how to control your weight with ease.

The one group says "It does not matter". The other group says "It is critically important". Another say 'You can't do anything about it." Off course I am talking about a major health controversy. Logically, when you find a large number of HEALTHY people to whom it does not matter, that is perfectly no issue. If you find a large number of people that are SICK (Obese) - then it might be an issue.

"However, if you find a lot of people that WERE sick and ARE now healthy - BECAUSE they changed something in their body; then there is a snake in the grass when conventional healthcare could not solve the problem.

Who would you believe? The ones that could never fix the weight problem (But made a LOT of money from sick people) - because they follow the standard route. Or the ones that taught you how to fix the problems - because they do not follow the standards of the first group."

There is one point that truly stands out above all else: The pH is of utmost critical issue in your body. In fact, it is so critical that your body has a number of different methods, even emergency methods, to control the pH of your blood and cells. Just to open the importance – your blood pH should be between 7.35 and 7.45. If it is more than 7.60 or lower than 7.20 you will be in a coma – or dead.

Fine, you cannot change the pH of your blood. You should not. Yes, all those who claim this are perfectly correct. However, since the real value on the pH scale between 7.2 and 7.6 is 0.4 – it means the alkalinity of your blood can vary a full 40 times in strength. Thus when I refer to a statement saying "Increase the alkalinity of your blood" I do not mean to make it 8.0. It is just to move away from the bottom edge and prompt it a little higher.

You will often find people claiming a statement like "To cure cancer, you need to reduce the acidity of your body. Cancer can't survive in an alkaline body." Yes, indeed that is true, but what pH do you need to change? How do you change that? Where do you measure it?

- What is pH?

pH (logarithmic Potential of Hydrogen) is a measurement of the concentration of the Hydrogen ions (H) ion in moles per liter. It expresses the acidity or alkalinity of a solution on a logarithmic scale on which 7 is neutral, lower values between 1 and 7 are acid, and higher values between 7 and 14 are alkaline. The pH level is important in every conceivable chemical and biological process. It is an easy method to indicate the hydrogen balance in a solution. At pH 7.0 we find a balance between Hydrogen ions = Hydroxide; that is called neutral.

The balanced Hydrogen atom is one Proton and one Electron. If the atom loses the electron, then it becomes Hydrogen Negative and if it gains an electron it is Hydrogen Positive. I know this is very simplified, but practical. One may ask why this lesson is important. It is because here is a big part of the story of why we get fat and other remain slim.

To write it out in mathematical will be 1.0×10^{-7} Moles. In decimal values the pH 2 will be 0.01, neutral pH 7.0 will be 0.0000001 and a pH of 9.5 will be written as 0.0000000095. Thus when we compare acidity from say pH 7.0; then a pH of 6.0 is ten times stronger acidity and 5.0 is hundred times stronger, 4.0 is a thousand times stronger acid. In practice the pH of various material will vary, but it is not important for us to be concerned about in this application of our bodies – which is water based.

There are many factors that affects a pH reading like pressure and temperature. For our body pH control we are always going to use the normal room and body temperatures.

One last issue on this stage, quite critical to remember. Our bodies are also electrical; and pH goes hand in hand with electrolytes. pH is married for life with Electrical Charge. Electrical charge not only affects the physical body, but it also reflects in the psychological. Ever wondered about the expression "He is a negative person"?

- How to measure pH?

Well, it is usually easy to go to a hospital, clinic or some doctors – let them do the work. But it is not really needed since you can do it yourself in seconds. You only need to buy pH strip papers, mostly available in pharmacies or Laboratory suppliers. Tear a strip off the package and dip it in the solution you wish to measure. The strip will change color, compare it to the color scale on the package and you are done. Easy. For our health and weight application, that is more than sufficient enough.

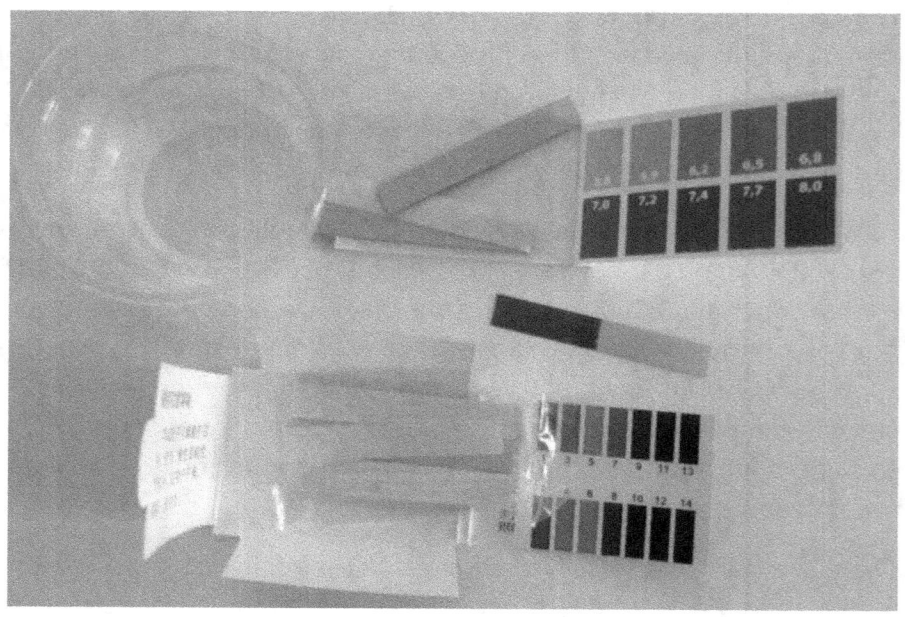

Easy to use pH strips, cheap at about US$ 2 for 100 test strips.

- What to measure?

You can only measure the pH of a solution, to measure solids is more complicated, but solution measurement is all we need. We need to measure our saliva in the mouth and our urine. If you sweat a lot, you can also measure that; though it is not really needed. There are a few issues to keep in mind when measuring. If you eat or drink something, it will immediately change your saliva pH, same is you even think of that nice cup of coffee the pH will change in the saliva. If you brush your teeth, it will affect the pH in your saliva for at least 30 minutes. If you drink a LOT of water, it will affect the pH of your urine. The same is also that the first bit of urine is actually remnants of the last time you urinated. If you are on kidney related medicine, it will affect your urine pH. Considering all of these there are a few guidelines. Always measure the pH in the same period and same conditions daily.

Keep a record of the time of day and conditions i.e. After Breakfast. You should build a data base of at least three measurements every day, same time, same conditions. This will give you a usable average. Readings of a few days - averaged out - is what you need to use.

For the saliva: Drink some water and rinse your mouth clean at the same time. Typically, just go on with your normal routines, preferably after eating. Make sure your mouth is not 'watering' because you think of that nice Black Forest cake of last Sunday. After not having any mouthwatering experiences, not eat or drink for at least 30 minutes, take a strip of pH paper and wet it with your saliva. Note the color changes, measure and record.

For the stomach: This is not a pleasant nor easy one. Do not do this three times a day, not even every day. Maybe once a week or when you really want to know. In general I would not recommend to do or measure this, because you will need to induce vomiting. IF (Not recommended) then you should measure when the stomach is as empty as possible. See the section in the appendix on how long some types of food remain in the stomach. You will need to only eat the fast digesting food that will pass out from stomach quickly for the whole day;

and drink pH 7.0 water all that day. In the evening or next morning – then have to induce vomiting, catch and measure.

There are other indications which I will explain later that is rather useful enough to determine the stomach pH condition.

In the beginning, I did this quite a lot (in the name of science), but it does have adverse effects on the stomach and esophagus.

For the Urine: Make a point of measuring three urine samples per day, one in the morning after waking up before eat or drink anything. This sample will usually be very acidic. The second test should be some time after lunch, try to keep similar period every day and the final one sometime between dinner and going to bed in evening. Always let a bit of urine out first before you capture the sample. Always makes sure your sample container is clean and dry to ensure better quality sample. Dip the paper strip, measure color and record.

To get the average of a few records, you add the numbers together and divide them by how many numbers were added together. As example if your morning reading is 6.3, midday is 7.2 and evening is 8.1, adding together is 21.6; divide by three will give you an average of 7.2 for the day.

- Important issues for pH.

There are a few things that will affect your pH values and it is critically important to keep this in mind.

The saliva is a glandular secretion, thus it is much affected by the internal pH of your body, blood and lymph; on top of that it is also greatly adopted by the various glands in your mouth. There is not too much you can do to affect the pH of the saliva. Thus, it is a good point to measure what is happening elsewhere.

The urine is a much more difficult issue. If you drink more water, the concentration of waste material in the urine will be lower and that will affect the pH value. If you drink too little water, your urine will be very acidic. Especially if you are losing weight which involves a lot more breaking down of cells and fats. Therefore, to get real usable values – you need to drink about same amount of water every day. Water, water, water and then whatever else you drink. I would suggest you stop drinking any other beverages.

Coffee for instance will make your whole system from mouth to urine more acidic, much more. Coke with all its fructose sugar will make your whole system acidic. If you remain on water only, try to drink same amounts of water throughout the day; that will then work in your favor to get reliable comparative pH reading from the urine. As example: drink a liter of water from waking up until lunch, half liter after lunch and half liter in evening; spread your water intake through this three parts of the day and try to remain as steady as possible. IF you do break this by for instance drinking coffee or beer etc. Then use some indicator to keep that in mind when you review your weekly controls. As example I will put a 'C' for coffee or 'B' for beer in my pH recoding block.

IMPORTANT: Try to maintain your volume of water intake. This is VERY important and even critical when weight is dropping. I do suggest you to make sure you never drink less than 1.5 liters of water per day, more is better. 'They' say you should drink one liter of water for every 25 kg of body weight. Even I live in the hot tropical Thailand that was not possible when my weight was 187 Kg! Now at 98 Kg it is still not possible. I just can't get to drink more than maybe 1.5 liters. You need to drink as much as what your body wants you to drink. The only single reason why water is of great importance here is that it makes the extraction and disposal of waste materials by the kidney and colon easier. Since you will lose weight, and cells will be broken down, it is advisable to provide enough funeral carriers (water) to dispose of the deceased cells.

- What should my body pH be?

Ahh, this is the critical question and one that most people do not understand. Your body is a biochemical factory. Various procedures and sections requires various pH levels. With that related, also various salinity and electrical charge levels.

Even here where it comes to the practical physical and real measureable they are disputed by medicine. A perfect balanced person in Mongolia will for instance have a stomach acidity of 1.3 where such will be an acidic problem for somebody living in Florida, USA. That said, in general the following are general indicators:

Your saliva should be around 7.0 to 7.5 if measured under above conditions.

Your stomach acid pH should vary between 1.5 and 3.5. Note: An important clue; in this program we will try to lift our stomach acid to vary between 3.0 and 4.0.

After the stomach, the acidic solution enters the Duodenum where the acidity is neutralized by bile and other digestive juices, including insulin. Then it will move through the small intestines which is about 6 meters long. There the content normal pH is about 6.0 up to 7.4. The blood will absorb whatever it needs from here. Finally, the stuff will pass through the colon where the pH will vary between 5.7 and 6.8; the more acidity is due to disposal of dead cells and other matter from the body.

The pH of your blood is very strictly controlled by a number of different organs and glands in the body. It has a very critical narrow band between 7.35 and 7.45. If it goes lower than 7.2 or higher than 7.6, your body will go into shock and you will enter a coma, any more changes and death is the result. BUT; do not fear, your body has plenty of reserves and many ways to control the critical blood pH. Cases of high alkalinity or acidity is rare.

The urine pH is not critical to the body in any manner. This is whatever the body dispose. However, it is a great indicator of what is happening inside your body. For us weight losers, this is the one item you wish to monitor – but you need to control everything else to get reliable readings here. Normally the urine of most people will vary somewhere between 6.0 in the morning and towards the evening it should go higher, even to 8.5.

AND THIS my friends are where you will need to set and control a target. Try to get your average urine for the day to be alkaline; above 7.0. This final indicator will then be your telltale that your body is 'alkaline'; though not exactly correct. But, it will only confirm there is no excess of acidity in your body, everything else is working on the pH level they need. A balanced fine-tuned body will not get sick. And will not gain excess weight.

- Symptoms of pH problems in body.

By no means are these symptoms only relevant to the pH – it could be an indicator of many other problems too. However, if you find you have more than five of the related symptoms; then you may accept your body is a little too alkaline or a little too acidic. As for this exercise in weight loss, our target is actually to get the body (blood and cells) a bit higher in alkaline state.

Testing the blood for pH is a bit more complicated than just cutting yourself and dipping a pH strip in it. It might work, but the fast oxidation of the blood will affect the result. In laboratories blood samples is usually handled in an enclosed sealed environment.

- Signs that your body might be too acidic:

Remember if your blood pH is lower than 7.35 you will feel sick, by 7.2 you will probably be in a coma and by 7.1 you will probably not be alive anymore. Thus the band for the blood pH is controlled very strictly by the body; at all times.

Regular coughing with no particular reason; though this could also be a shortage of calcium.

Irregular Heart Beat.

Your pulse rate will be higher for no apparent reason. A good pulse rate at rest should be varying between 58 and 65.

If your body was in high acidic state for a long time, you will probably find an excessive growth of skin tags and warts.

The skin will be dry, often itching.

You might sleep, but will not have a deep rest. At all times it seems the brain just can't switch off.

Muscular weakness, feeling of tiredness in muscles all the time.

You will probably feel a constant slight nausea.

Your sweat will have an acidic smell.

Have a constant anxiety feeling, like a dark looming threat.

Frequent gasping for oxygen, feels like not enough oxygen in blood.

That also leads to holding breath – you may not be able to hold your breath past 30-seconds.

- Signs that your body might be too alkaline:

The body is not able to absorb sufficient minerals from intestines; thus in general you will have all signs of insufficient mineral supplements.

Low level of potassium in blood.

Cramps in calves, heart rate irregular.

Low calcium in blood.

A twitching in the face, especially under left eye.

Skin will be oilier, even a problem with acne.

Hyperventilating.

Arthritis.

Easy fungal and bacterial infections, candida, athlete's foot, etc.

Many allergies, often manifesting in blocking sinus cavities.

Abnormal bone growth, like spurs.

Low Thyroid activity.

Calcium being deposited on bones rather than performing other functions.

- How to change the pH?

To change the pH of some parts in your body is easier than people think. Off course 'they' will tell you it is not possible. Well, I tell you 'they' are wrong. There are a few important issues: Remember you can't really control the pH of your blood – not by any large factor through your digestive system anyway.

By changing the food you eat and whatever you drink; you will have a major direct effect on the stomach and intestines, from there it will then also have a minor effect on the blood and the rest of the body. We want to achieve a less acidic stomach. That is to reduce the breakdown of food; reduce the demand for food through hunger feelings and through all of this – to reduce the requirements and production of insulin.

Following that is the final part of the alkalizing of the body; to push the blood pH level up, just a by a small notch or two. Get over the 7.40 mark is perfect, and there is an easy way to test it. BUT, there are ways in which you will feel the difference and you will know when it happens. The wonderful items which you can easily measure then; is the drop of your weight.

Besides the digestive system and some mineral concepts, there is one way in which you can directly change the pH of your blood in as little as 5 minutes – breathing routines.

- Stomach pH.

By far the easiest way to reduce the acidity of your stomach is by consuming anti-acids; in particular Baking Soda. To do this procedure, the best option I can suggest is the one big teaspoon of baking soda in a 600 ml of water bottle, consumed throughout the day – but NOT within 30 minutes before or after your meal(s). You do not want to strip all the acid from your stomach when you eating – the acid is important to digest your food (which we do not worry about too much) AND to digest the minerals – which we DO worry about very much.

However, you have to keep that little bacteria called *H. Pyloric* in mind. Due to a lack of knowledge there, I did make a mistake here. For a few months (December 2016 until mid-February 2017) these things in my stomach exploded. They bumped my stomach acidity right to Uranus; leaving me with a stomach pH of 6.2 and some days even as high as 7.0.

I strongly recommend you not to let the stomach acidity go higher than 4.0 or maybe 4.2. It may take more time to reach the changes inside the rest of your body, but that would be preferable than a fast change; and H. Pylori explosion.

Though the baking soda is an easy fast way to increase the alkalinity; I rather suggest you follow a more natural and slower way. See later about food to change the pH, but I will suggest you consider the path of fresh squeezed lemon juice. About 50 ml first thing every morning. Lemon remains acidic (pH about 2.2) until in the stomach; however, the friendly enzymes in your stomach will convert the acidic lemon juice to a very valuable alkaline based juice (pH about 7.8) by the time it passes into the duodenum.

When the stomach pH goes higher than 4.0 that little valve that prevents reflux into the esophagus loses its functionality. Food get up the wrong way, you start getting heartburn aka GERD. The worse is that the bacteria are now getting dominant in your stomach and whenever you eat anything even slightly acidic; there is an unwanted bio-chemical reaction taking place.

Such reaction between acid and alkali usually results in foam. Such foam will cause air bubbles. And the air bubbles will be hurting you. Ahh, the same reason babies cry when they have air locked in the stomach, when they burp it out, they are happily relaxed. When this issue is getting worse, you will find that food gets stuck at the lower esophagus valve. It simply cannot get into your stomach, because the stomach is filled with foam and under slight pressure.

Even more bad news is that whatever you eat, and whatever does reach to your stomach – cannot get out to the Duodenum and intestines because that valve only allows acidic and broken down (fermented) material through. At one time I could not even get water through. Suffered for two days, started to dehydrate.

The good news is this: As long as you know what the symptoms are, and are ready for it – it is very easy and relative quick to fix.

I do admit that my stomach went suddenly over alkaline because of this *H. Pyloric* bacteria exploding. And I do state that it was damn uncomfortable. It was also worry some, especially since I did not immediately know what was going on.

CRITICAL ADVICE: Do not consume alkaline changing substances for more than 2 months. After two months, let the acidity of your stomach rule for a while. My mistake was that I went for alkaline stomach (my target was around 6.0) for too long. Better to use the stepping routing. Six weeks alkalizing stomach, three weeks normal acidic.

So how do we get this bug under control again?

Easy, just get your stomach back into acid state. For me that was difficult because the pH has been too high for too long, thus the bugs were in control. I therefore needed to give help from outside.

The very good remedy is Apple Cider Vinegar; raw, unfiltered. About 2 spoons full in some water before every meal. Unfortunately for me, I could not stand the taste of Apple Cider at all, not in the raw pure form. However, I love cooking with it and there I love the taste.

The second option will cost a little money, for me it was absolute worth it. Even though I had a long search in Thailand to find this kind of product. This is VERY powerful. It is called Betaine HCL. The stomach acid is Hydrochloric Acid (HCL). So this Betaine HCL is a direct supplement for exactly the same acid in a capsule form. You need to start off with one capsule before eating any protein kind of meal. If it does not solve the problem, then go up to two capsules. Some people even went as high as 9 capsules. What you need to look out for is a slight burning hot feeling in the stomach region – that is the point where the acid is too much. From there you step one capsule down. In time right back to one and finally zero. When buying this kind of capsules, I suggest you get one bottle with more than 600 mg caps and one with only 200 mg caps. I use the higher dosage when I eat protein, the lower dosage (usually in combination with enzymes and other) I use when eating a non-protein meal.

The third option, and this one finally worked quickly for me, is to go for pre-fermented food. This is often called Super Foods, and that is not an overstatement. I am talking of foods like Sauerkraut and other similar naturally fermented foods – which you should make yourself. Though in many countries/cities you can buy. Why I suggest you make yourself is so that you can know exactly what goes into that bottle, and that it is pure organic. This kind of foods can be made from just about any vegetable. From fruit also, though fruit will be sugar based and form alcohol rather that the desired lacto bacteria. You can google "Fermented Foods" and/or Sauerkraut. On my Facebook and website I will place a few links and recipes of my own.

Lastly, not so effective when you have a big problem; but more when the problem is reducing and you find the acid levels are getting near normal. In particular, this is also very helpful when you do not have a problem with the stomach acidity lost out of control, but rather just a bit of reflux or heartburn. Drink a freshly squeezed lemon juice. First thing in the morning. One every day, can take with no more than same volume measure of water and adding a small pinch of Himalayan salt is a perfect cure/maintenance.

The moment you add acid back into your stomach, you will suffer for a day or two from lots of foam. Typically foam vomiting.

Please do take care when sleeping since this might push right up to your throat and even over into your lungs. A rude chocking awakening I do not wish you to experience. Therefore, I learned to sleep a few days with my chest and shoulders at a relative steep inclining angle to keep the throat above the stomach level.

Ok, after a few days of foamy chemical reaction in your stomach, things will quiet down, stomach will become more acidic and you can get back to enjoying every bite of whatever you wish to eat; within the parameters of your diet. During and short after this 'killing the bugs foamy period' you probably will notice your stool being of near black color. It is actually a very dark green. That is H. Pyloric losing the war.

Thus do not fear (like I did) that there is blood from internal bleeding in my feces and run off to the hospital! This can last for up to a week.

IF you do go for a more alkaline stomach, I suggest you not let it go higher than 4.0 or maybe 4.2. Do maintain a limited time of no more than 6 weeks per session. Do not go for long time to allow bacteria and fungi to get out of control.

The moment you find it somewhat difficult to swallow food, especially meat, chicken or fish and if somewhat dry meat; or the moment you find protein like cream or milk makes you feel nausea – stop the alkalinity process and get back into acid forming food or drinks like lemon juice or even real coffee.

- Breathing.

This is the only method in which you can directly change the pH of your blood, within limits. The body will not allow the blood pH to go higher than 7.43 regardless how much you breathe. By this method you are not only changing the pH with all that advantages, but you enrich your blood with oxygen and that will have a massive amount of other beneficial advantages in your body, brain and spiritual realms. I used a similar technique in the beginning, but later learned about the extremely effective *Wim Hof Method*. You can Google or YouTube search for some of his videos.

Basically the routine is three cycles of three steps each:

Get your body in a comfortable position, yoga lotus position if you can, or sit upright on the bed IF you can. Else you can even lie down on your back with head on pillow. It is not serious what your position is, as long as you are comfortable. Although, an upright position will increase the required effects. As you progress in losing weight and better breathing, try to get up until you can sit in Lotus yoga position.

Start by breathing deep into your lungs, as much as you can. Breathe in at medium or normal speed. Then breathe out as quickly as possible, as much as you can. Repeat for about 30 times. The right term is 'hyperventilating'. All the time concentrate on what is happening in your body, ignore the light headedness when you start of first time. Keep the whole cycle's rhythmic, flowing like a calm ocean wave; deep in, and deep out.

After the last breath, exhale to normal level (not forcing everything out) and close your system down, do not inhale for as long as you can. You should be able to hold out for about 2 minutes. Then when you really need to inhale, take two deep breaths in, hold the second one in your lungs and push the air towards your head/brain. You will literally feel the rush through your body. Exhale slowly and start the whole routine over again. The second cycle you should be able to hold your breath somewhere around 3 minutes. After the third cycle, you could even reach 5 minutes. In all, this routine should take about 15 minutes. Three session of 5 minutes each in a row.

Because of prior techniques, I used breathing in a similar way; I do find sometimes that I may go in a spiritual state, even while on the breathing step. One day I reached six and half minutes before breathing air; I think I only pumped the air about eighteen times. An amazing experience it certainly is.

Do this three-cycle routine twice a day. Best is just after waking up, before eating or drinking anything, on an empty stomach. Do the second session anytime late afternoon or evening, BUT not less than 2 hours before sleeping time; else it might affect your falling asleep. You can do more sessions per day, though I would not recommend it from the beginning. Better start with one set per day then after a week you can do second set per day.

What exactly is happening in your body is quite interesting. First with the rapid deep breaths you clear the lungs of carbon dioxide and other gasses like nitrogen, fill them with more of the normal 21% oxygen rated air. By the way of passing; if you can do this during daytime in a forest or densely vegetation area; it is much better because air there are usually higher in oxygen (up to 22.5%) and lower in nitrogen. Then the blood can absorb more oxygen and release more of the waste carbon dioxide. More oxygen rich blood is of lighter red color. The blood can thus transport more oxygen throughout your body, which increases your metabolic processes as well as regulate cell functions.

The time you stop breathing, that is the time your brain will kick into a strange mode; I find it akin to a deep meditation. During that time the brain re-establish communications with the rest of your body.

Then, when you hold the next deep breath, it forces energy right through your body. For me, each and every time, I can literally feel the gulf of energy rippling through every part from head to toe.

After the second cycle, I feel energized. After the third I am almost ready to tackle Mount Everest. This does not only affect your physical body – but also your subconscious and conscious parts in the brain, every organ and every cell.

AND: Because of the higher oxygen content, this routine directly affects the fluid between every cell in your body. It makes your blood and cellular fluid that required little bit more alkaline; directly and quickly.

So, what does this has to do with weight loss?

Surprisingly a heck of a lot. How does this sounds to you, "Breathe oxygen in, Breathe fat out". Yes, if you breathe more, deeper and enrich your oxygen level in the blood; you will literally lose fat from your body, through your lungs! Guess why I said 'you do not need to do lots of exercises' in this program? Doing this breathing routine is a lot easier and very effective for us obese people.

You see, human fat cells store large heavy triglyceride (a type of fat in the blood) which is made up of carbon, hydrogen and oxygen. These atoms are broken into smaller molecules and released through oxidation (High oxygen in the blood) and when that happens, fat is burned off.

Here is a lesser known chemical fact. Remember when I talked about what pH is? It is related to the positive and negative ions of Hydrogen.

So what happens when you have a higher level of oxygen in the blood, combined with the normal constituents between your body cells; they re-absorb the hydrogen. When the Hydrogen is gone, the fat breaks down into carbon dioxide (CO_2). Scientists from the University of New South Wales in Australia did some math. When 10 kg of fat is oxidized, 8 kg leave the body through the lungs as hydrogen and CO_2. The remaining 2 kg becomes water. To effectively burn the 10 kg of fat from the body, you will need to use 30 kg of oxygen. During a normal slow day, you lose around 200 gram of fat through the normal average 22,000 times you let a breath out.

Besides this new knowledge; a higher level of oxygen in the blood makes it possible for the body in increase metabolism; and that needs more energy. First the body will take from the blood sugars what it needs; if there is still lots of free oxygen, then the body will start to utilize the stored fats.

Through this breathing routines you can lose an extra one to one and half kilograms per month; and generate a lot of other healthy advantages for your body on the side.

In addition to all the weight loss advantages, there is another important value. Higher oxygen in the blood helps to fight undesirable bacteria and fungi; especially if you have a leaky gut syndrome.

- Signs and Monitoring.

You will need to learn reading and listening to your body.

Your body needs to learn communication.

We tend to ignore the most important thing in our existence – our bodies. It is there and unless we are in pain; we seldom really think and take note of things. Nails grow and needs to be trimmed, hair the same, but did you notice the speed of growth? Do you notice the shine and health in your hair and nails? How about the skin of your feet sole and heels? There are a number of things you need to watch in your body.

All the time make notes, be it mental or on paper. Notice your skin, eyes, urine, feces, lips, nails, earwax ... How often do you go to the toilet? All of these are important for your general health and when losing weight – it is even more critical.

By no means possible is this list of things I monitor the full spectrum, neither can I even think of all the smallest details to note. This is just a general overview, of what I do all the time, by that I mean daily or at least once a week.

Remember, one of the changes I made is the pH of my body? That is most directly visible on the skin. For a number of years I had quite a lot of 'skin-tags', a few warts and moles all over my body. Used many types of chemicals to burn them off. Earlier last year I read in a medical paper that those are usually an indicator of high acidic pH on the skin and in the muscles of the body. The suggestion was to change the body pH a little upwards, closer to the 7.40 mark. Only problem is that they did not expand on how to do it.

Anyway, when I went on the diet programs and there did change my body pH – amazingly; my skin tags and warts reduced. Last time I used acid was a bit over a year ago and then my darling had to cover some 140 tags on my back side, and I did about the same number on the front. A few months later I still had remnants of more than 80. I know this because I went to a dermatologist for a quote to laser burn them! Some US$ 32,000! Funny thing, when I thought to write about this here – I have only 18 left – and their sizes are reducing anyway!

The lesson: Watch your skin for potential problems. Your skin tells you a lot about the pH of your body and also about the minerals present in your body. As soon as your body starts developing a mineral issue – it WILL show up in your skin, hair and nails.

Urine: There is one thing people fail to take note off. You must, very critically important. No, you do not need to catch a sample and run off to a laboratory every time, just look and note. How does it smell (from normal distance), what is the color, does it burn when you take the leak, are there signs of fatty oil floating, is there little pieces that looks like blood or strings? Maybe it has some milky looking particles. All of these are indicators that something is happening in your body. As a matter of interest; the Urine is affected within less than one hour after an event in the body. Anything in your digestive system, blood, lymph, liver, kidneys, lungs, heart – all of your body is reflected in your urine; quickly. Even before you will consciously know something is wrong.

Eye: This is a more long term mirror on your body. Everything that is happening anywhere in the body (related to nerve or sensors) are reflected in the iris of the eye. There is an extreme accurate diagnostic tool know as Iridology where a practitioner can read your physical history and even tell you what problems are busy developing in your body. Though I did study the basics of this from Dr. Bernard Jensen of Boulder, Colorado in the USA – I do not practice it and my knowledge after some 25 years has gone quite lost.

One of the reasons I went on this severe diet plans was that I took a good long look in a mirror; about May 2016 – and I was quite surprised to see problems developing. Even signs of potential cancer that I did not realize. Just small red to dark red spots. I realized that I need to act quickly, red can still be reverted (healed) when they get black it is mostly beyond healing. You can easily get some free diagrams from the internet and use those for a very rough superficial diagnosis. Should you find there are potential problems, I would urge you to go visit a practicing Iridologist for proper diagnosis. In the meantime – get on a suitable diet for whatever region you find there may be a problem i.e. kidney, liver, thyroid, etc.

However, that is not all. The white of the eye is telling you about condition of liver and kidneys, blood pressure, viral infections and many more. Excessive sodium deposits is reflected in the eye.

The Eye is a window to your whole body.

Nails: Beyond the normal skin-hair-nail issues; there is a whole series of diagnosis that can be read from the nails. These are not reflecting short term issues, it takes many months or even years to develop the indicators on your nails.

Feces (Stool): Hmm, some people told me not to use the better explaining word . . . Anyway, when you made the long drop you also need to see what is coming out. The color, structure and whatever else is noticeable. As one example: I may eat a cucumber on Monday morning and then look how long it takes until the seed is in the toilet. That tells me what the average speed of my digestive system is. As with urine, you do not need to take a sample and go to your microscope. Just a cursory glance before you flush is usually good enough. Color tells you what you ate and how effective the intestines were absorbing whatever they needed. Density tells you very much about your water consumption.

Your body talks to you through the urine, through your eye, your own tongue, your skin. Listen and react.

The Urine: That tells you what is happening in your blood.

The sh . . . I mean stool: That tells you what is happening in your digestive system.

The skin and nails: tells Talk to you about the state of minerals and oils in your body.

The Eyes: Tells you what is happening in your nervous system (and much more advanced).

- Diet.

I said it a few times, and I will keep on saying it until you are overflown with the concept. Cut out ALL sugar, 100%. Start to force your body to retrieve the fatty storage for energy.

Reduce – preferably cut out completely – all grain products, especially the highly refined ones like white rice, white wheat. And especially those that are most likely Genetic Modified like corn, wheat, soy and canola, etc.

Consume no acidic forming food – and absolutely no coffee. Try to remain with food that are rather alkaline forming.

The actual pH of food when measured in fresh state, is not how it will change inside your body. For example; milk is usually alkaline (7.8 to 8.5) but after digestion it will be more acidic like 5.5 to 6.0. Lemon juice is very acidic, as low as 1.6 but after it passes through the stomach it will have an alkaline effect of the body. Laboratory technicians can determine how foods will react inside the body by incinerating the food to ash. The mineral content of the ash is then measured for the pH; that indicates how such food item will affect the pH in your body. However, these are just general indicators. Each and every product will be greatly affected by the environment where such is produced. The type of soil used to grow fruits and vegetables.

The following I will list two groups of foods: Alkaline and Acidic forming. However, do remember: This is final effect – AFTER the stomach and digestion. Many of these alkaline effect items will actually be acidic and initially produce acid in the stomach.

One excellent example is my beloved lemon. Now that I need to make my stomach more acidic, but do not want my whole system to get back to a very acidic state, this is the best to consume. A fresh lemon juiced first thing in the morning. It does make more acid in the stomach, but has an alkaline effect on the rest of the body.

- Here is a basic list of the more Alkaline forming foods; in alphabetical order.

Almonds, Apples, Apricots, Artichokes, Arugula, Asparagus, Avocado, Baking soda, Banana, Beet, Bell pepper, Blackberry, Blueberry, Broccoli, Brussels sprouts, Cabbage, Cantaloupe, Carob, Carrots, Cashews, Cauliflower, Cayenne pepper, Celery, Cherry, Chestnuts,

Chive, Cilantro, Citrus, Collard green, Cucumber, Currant, Dandelion, Dewberry, Eggplant, Endive, Flax seeds, Garlic, Ghee, Ginger, Ginseng, Grapefruit, Grapes, Green beans, Hemp seed oil, Herbs (leafy green), Honey (some), Kale, Kelp, Kiwifruit, Kohlrabi, Leeks, Lemons, Lentils, Lettuces, Limes, Loganberry, lotus root, Mango, Mushrooms, Mustard green, Nectarine, Nutritional yeast, Oats, Okra, Olive, Onion, Orange, Papaya, Parsley, Parsnip, Passion fruit, Peach, Pear, Peas, Pepper, Pineapple, Potato, Pumpkin, Pumpkin seed, Quinoa, Radishes, Raisin, Raspberries, Rutabaga, Sea vegetables, Seaweed, Sesame seed, Soy sauce, Spirulina, Sprouts, Squashes, Strawberry, Sunflower seeds, Sweet corn (fresh), Sweet potato, Tahini, Tangerine, Taro root, Turnip, Turnip greens, Vegetable juices, Watercress, Watermelon.

- This is a basic list of more Acidic forming foods; in alphabetical order.

Adzuki beans, Aged cheese, Alcohol, Almond oil, Amaranth, Balsamic vinegar, Barley, Basmati Rice, Beef, Black-eyed peas, Brazil nuts, Breads, Brown rice, Brown sugar, Buckwheat, Butter, Canola oil, Casein, Chard, Chicken, Chutney, Cocoa, Coconut, Coffee, Cottage cheese, Cow milk, Cranberry, Cream, Curry, Dates, Dry fruit, Egg whites, Fava beans, Figs, Fish, Flour (white), fried foods, Fructose, Fruit juices, Game meat, Garbanzo beans, Gelatin, Goat cheese, Goat milk, Goose, Grape seed oil, Green peas, Guava, Hazelnuts, Honey (some), Hops, Ketchup, Kidney beans, Lamb, Lard, Lima beans, Lobster, Malt, Maple syrup, Milk, Millet, Mollusks, Mussels, Mustard, Mutton, Nutmeg, Oat bran, Olives (pickled), Pasta, Pastry, Peanuts, Pecans, Pheasant, Pickles, Pine nuts, Pinto beans, Pistachio seeds, Plum, Pomegranate, Popcorn, Pork, Processed cheese, Prunes, Red beans, Rhubarb, Rye, Seafood, Semolina, Sesame oil, Shell fish, Soy milk, Soybean, Spinach, Squid, String beans, Sunflower oil, Table salt, Tapioca, Tofu, Tomatoes, Turkey, Veal, Walnuts, Wheat, White beans,

White bread, White rice, White vinegar, Whole wheat foods, Wine, Yeast, Yogurt, Zucchini.

- Drink lots of water.

Whatever you do and however you feel – you have to drink lots of water. The more, the better. If you do not drink at least 1.5 liters of water per day, your urine will never go alkaline. Since you are in the process of eliminating fat cells, those has to be disposed out from the body. But in the breaking down part, the cells release a lot of acidic material; same as when you exercise – lactic acids. That is disposed of via the kidneys and urinary system. If the urinary system remains very acidic with all this additional material passing through – the changes of you developing kidney stones are very high. THAT my dear reader I assure you is the one pain you do not want to experience. I had an 8 mm stone that took nearly two weeks to pass through. The suffering was beyond anything I could ever explain. Yes, even women say they will rather have ten natural births than one more kidney stone. So do drink a LOT of water.

- Alkaline water – Baking Soda.

For the sake of alkalinity and also for a number of other reasons, you can drink Baking Soda, or if you can get the preferred better natural version Nacholite, in your water. At the beginning I made my water a pH of 9.0 which was way too alkaline. Yes, when my weight started dropping, it went fast. Too fast. But later on I also had some other problems, like the struggle to get my stomach acidic again.

Do NOT use alkaline water for more than 6 weeks in one session.

I recommend you take a bottle of somewhere between 600 and 800 ml of water in the morning, add a heaped teaspoon of baking soda to the bottle and shake well. Ideal pH around 8.0 for this water. Keep the bottle in your fridge, it is good to have this water near freezing, or just forming a little ice flakes in the bottle. Drink from that bottle in such way that you finish it over a 12-hour period, throughout the day, before sleep. A bonus effect here: you will be pleasantly surprised on how good your stomach and head feels after the third day. Do not drink any of this water for at least 30 minutes before and after your meal(s). Do not eat anything within 30 minutes either side of drinking Baking Soda water. You can drink any other water, pH between 7.0 and 7.5 as much as you possible can at any time. Make sure your water pH is above 7.0 at all times.

NOTE AGAIN: Do not use alkaline water when you are on the High Fat Diet. With that diet you will need all possible acid in your stomach to process the food efficiently.

Chapter 3 - Potato Only Diet.

Purpose: To lose weight, reduce the body craving for foods, especially sugars and to reduce the volume of food per meal. To get your body off the three plus meals a day concept. To get your meal times set in preparation for the later coming diets. Off course, the loss of a few kilograms of weight is a great bonus, no better motivation.

Yes, indeed there is a potato only diet – and it is working. Well, at least it did work for me, very well. However, when on this diet one lose a certain amount of weight, but then you reach a plateau where it is difficult to break through.

The interesting thing with this is that officially the recommended amount of potato is way beyond what I could ever reach. Potatoes are a weak form of Carbohydrates. A fist size potato has about 15 grams of carbohydrates, which includes about 0.8 gram of sugars. (Remember how much sugar your body needs? Five potatoes per day will give it all the sugar it needs; about one teaspoon full).

Although there are a small amount of carbs and sugars, it does not spike the insulin. Maybe because the other ingredients and minerals hides the sugar? This is one of the good reasons to start your diet program with the potato only diet. The most important part of this program I followed is based on a Low-Carb-High-Fat diet; then why am I talking of a Potato only diet?

The answer is simple, with many facets. Potatoes makes you feel full. It does not spike the secretion of insulin. There is a slow wave like increase of insulin when eating potato. It is monotonous, plain boring, but the feeling in the stomach is very OK. However, after a few meals it becomes boring, makes it much easier to skip meals and get to the two or One Meal A Day routine. Above all of this, it helps to 'educate' and force your body to retrieve some of that stored fats and convert it to whatever the body needs.

Of this I am not totally sure; but for myself it seems the potato had a digestive system cleansing effect too. Take note of the color and odor of your stool on daily basis.

The potato diet does not work for everyone. If you go on this diet, you should see results within the first 3 or 4 days. If after two weeks you did not lose more than a kilogram, then you are probably in the group that will not lose weight with a potato diet – or you are not eating only potato. However, you can still use this diet for the purpose of getting off the food addiction and reach the point where your meals (and stomach) become smaller and reduced eating volume in the whole day.

The best and most effective way to go on this diet is to eat only water-boiled potatoes. How much or how many is up to you. The general consensus is that to maintain your current body weight, you need to eat one fist size potato for every ten kilograms (2 pounds) of weight, per day. For me it meant I needed to eat 18 potatoes per day! Any less than that and the weight will drop.

To be more practical;

Breakfast - eat as many boiled potatoes as you need to make your stomach full.

Lunch – eat as many boiled potatoes as you need to make your stomach full.

Dinner – eat as many boiled potatoes as you need to make your stomach full.

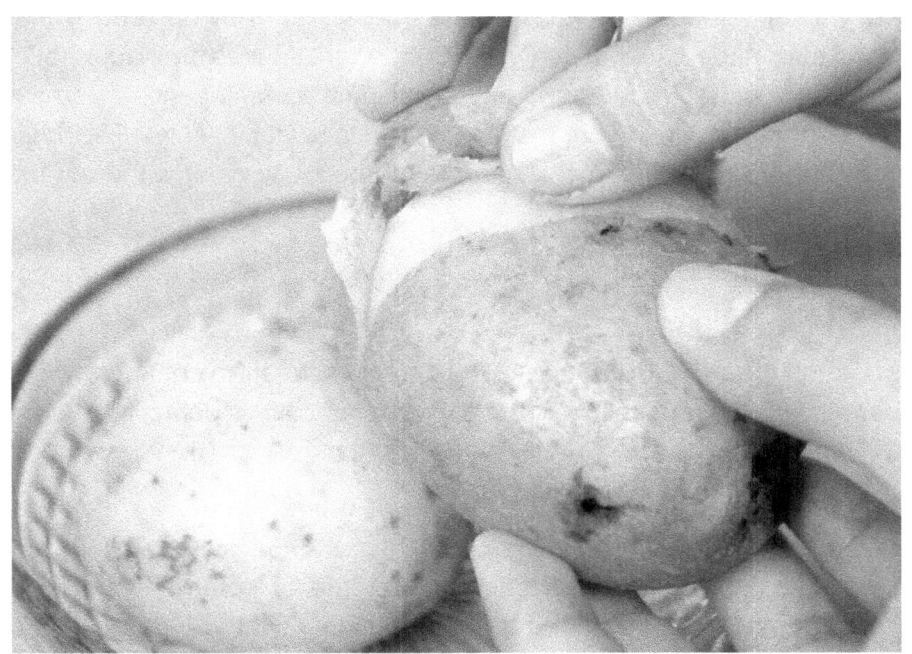

The purest form of Potato Diet only is the fastest to lose weight.

Although you can use some taste enhancers; for faster effects – eat only boiled, steamed, baked or grilled potato. A very small amount of fried potato is ok for maybe twice a week. NOTHING else with it. Boring as hell, effective as heavens.

Then after a few days, you start shifting the meals. Make breakfast later in the morning. Make dinner earlier in the evening or late afternoon. Eventually cut lunch out completely. Try to reach potato breakfast around 10h00 in the morning and potato dinner around 16h00 (4 pm) in the afternoon.

Drink as much water as you can manage; as long as you do not drown.

There are just a few small points to remember.

DO NOT EAT ANYTHING ELSE DURING THIS DIET; PERIOD.

Even eating salads, leafy herbs, taste enhancers; they do reduce the weight loss speed. Any such nice tasty stuff causes the automatic secretion of insulin by the pancreas; awaiting the coming meal. You do NOT want any spike in your insulin levels. None at all. Why? Because when there is higher insulin in the blood, the body can't withdraw fat from the storages.

To say it in a nice positive way; "You can eat anything you wish, as long as it is a boring potato".

By potato I mean POTATO. Yes, you can substitute the common white tuber also for the red, yellow or even black potato. This potato diet does NOT include the Sweet Potato which contains 40 to 100 times more sugars. You do not want the sugars!

If you break this rule by eating other things, especially any form of protein, grain or sugars with or near the time of potato – whatever potato you ate WILL be added to your body fat. That you do not want to happen, so stay away from other food. If living with other people and often being exposed to wonderful aromas coming from the kitchen; make sure you eat your fill with potato before they start cooking. A full stomach is usually not a good appetizer. Or go for a walk.

Eat nothing else with the potatoes.

Absolutely NO Protein and NO Sugars; not even honey or shop bought sauces like ketchup, mayonnaise, etc. You can make your own, ensuring that you know exactly what goes in conforms to your diet plan.

Nothing else than water in between the meals.

Let me add an important part here; eat nothing else with the potato diet. Yes, one might be tempted to use a lot of herbs or vegetables – after all they do not make you fat. Here, that is the absolute wrong idea. The moment you eat other things with the potato, your body snaps onto that for its nutrition and the potato goes to weight gain. Such will spike your insulin and body stops using the fat for energy. In best case scenario, you will find yourself on a weight loss plateau; no more dropping of weight. In the worst case scenario, all the efforts you did until then is lost and you will need to start all over again.

Yes, this diet is not a real enjoyable one, but it is potentially very effective. The good news is that later on you can go on a different kind of diet and enjoy a tasty life while losing weight; fast and effective.

OK, I yield, cooked potato-only is a real punishment. So I did cheat half way. I did not eat any other foods, but I did add some stuff to make my potato more consumable. You can cheat (yourself) but it does reduce the weight loss tempo a bit. I accepted that and lived with it. Hey a kilo a week is still better than nothing. But ten kilograms a month is a hell of a big pleasure to experience. It only depends on you yourself.

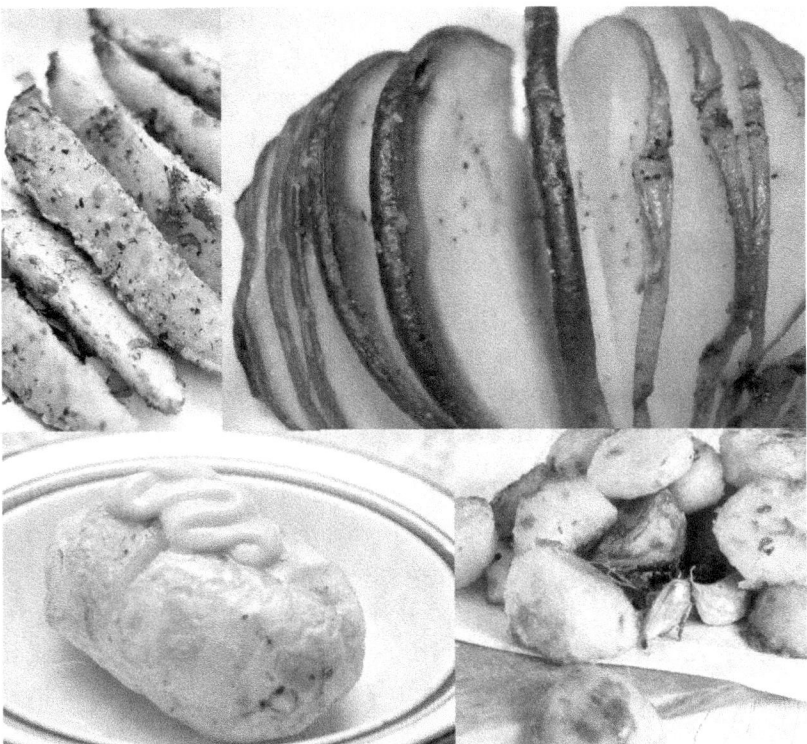

There are literally hundreds of ways to cook potato – suitable for this diet. You can use Google and search for 'Potato Cooking / Potato Baking / Potato Steaming / etc.'

You can add all sorts of herbs and spices. I used salt, freshly ground pepper, chili, oregano, thyme, parsley, turmeric (Excellent spice to add), garlic, etc. These will not affect the weight loss; well not much.

In itself these things does not make you gain any weight. But, this is the crucial secret. It does make your mouth water, secretes saliva. And that on its own do activate insulin production, and increased insulin in the intestines will become increased insulin in the blood; that will cause storage of nutrients in the cells and prevents fat from being extracted. You definitely do not want increased insulin levels; thus do not eat the most wonderful taste enhancers with your potatoes.

Many times I will eat a potato spud with a bit of butter – the emphases on LITTLE BIT. Like quarter a teaspoon per meal. Sometimes I will make a potato salad; boiled potato, a LITTLE bit of my own homemade mayonnaise and mustard, some fresh parsley, dill and/or coriander. Sometimes I may cook the potato in curry, quite nice. Make a mash and bake a dried herb crust on top in the oven. A cooked potato, lightly coated in butter and heavily spiced with hot chili and some oregano – well that quickly satisfies any appetite.

And yes, French fries aka Chips is also OK. But once or twice a week and then half your normal portion. Use unsaturated oils like Olive, Avocado, Sesame or Palm oil to fry your potato. Same for other cooking like pan-fried. Though, your weight loss tempo will definitely be slower!

Do remember; do not eat anything else during this stage of your program. If you really can't resist it anymore, please just try to hold out for at least 6-hours before and after eating any potato. Stay away from cruciferous vegetables. During your break month from the potato diet, it is highly recommended that you eat a large number of these to replenish minerals. For some reason, I do not understand exactly why, vegetables like broccoli, cauliflower, Brussels sprouts, cabbage, and Pok Choy seems to terminate the potato effects. I am still trying to find the reasons.

Definitely a BIG no to any meat, grain, fatty or sweet product. This includes even honey. If you break this rule, your insulin will spike and you will go back to day one of suffering. Rather wait until you get to the High Fat diet later on.

Oh, there are three more items you can eat with your potato, no unwanted effect. Well maybe a bit of air. You can eat onions, garlic and carrots. Remember, add some onions to your potato; not potato to your onions! Much more potato, some onion. A few (or plenty) cloves of garlic can only do good, not only will it help cleaning the blood, may even increase weight loss speed.

The same is valid for your general eating of herbs; add a little herb to your potato is OK but do not add potato to your herbs! In effect this means like a teaspoon of green chopped herbs or quarter of a teaspoon of dried herbs.

This is a full time diet, your body will get all it needs from the potato for a short period and the rest it will retrieve from the stored material. The important part is that potato does not spike the insulin. Take care not to put anything with sugar on your potato. That includes sweet mayonnaise, ketchup, etc.

Try to keep this diet going for between 6 weeks and two months. Depends on your weight and how strict you are in the potato only eating; you may lose as little as 2 kg or as much as 20 kg; it is entirely up to you. Then you need to change the diet altogether or step off for a month to eat a variety of other foods in order to build you vitamins and minerals in the body. After a month, you can get back on the potato diet. Yes, I am aware of people that went on potato only for a year; and lost like 70 kg. I am just concerned about the other functions in your body that needs minerals; thus a prolonged diet of only potato will deplete some of your minerals and vitamins – that is not a good thing.

Normally I would say "Do not peel your potato" because much of the nutrition is just below the skin. Unless you are sure your potatoes are cultivated in a complete organic manner; or by yourself – then do peel your shopped potato. This is to reduce the exposure to modern agriculture and preservation methods with their chemicals.

Always monitor your weight and the energy you feel through your day. It is a good practice to sleep at least 7 hours at night and take a nice half to one-hour nap around midday. You will probably be surprised to find you have more energy on day to day basis and you will find you sleep better at night.

I suggest you not keep strict on this diet for more than two months per session. At some time, your weight loss will reach a plateau; no more reduction. For me it was twice when I reached a loss of about 20 kg. Do not fear or worry, that is where we want to be, next phase to start.

Besides the main long time potato diet, during the other forms of diet like High Fat there are times your body just tells you "STOP the fat". Then it is easy to revert back to potato only for a day or two. However – do maintain the two or one meal a day and still maintain the not eating anything else for at least 6 hours before and after eating potato.

The potato will normally take between 45 minutes and 90 minutes to pass through your stomach. It will linger around 6 to 8 hours in your intestines and more than 2 hours in your colon. If you do drink a lot of water, your toilet visit for a long-drop will be an easy, soft and comfortable one; once a day.

Finally, a piece of wonderful news. After a week or so you will find the craving for food is missing; you will even find the 'want' to eat those nice pieces of steak or Black forest cake is no more. Suddenly, tasting anything sugary will make you feel like vomiting! This then is the proof you are on the way to reach whatever target you set for your ultimate dream weight.

Now it is time to answer a technical question: "What does the potato give to me?"

Nutritional values of potato varies between the different cultivars as well as the agricultural conditions in which they are cultivated. Officially a 250 gram meal of the normal white potato contains about:

1,000 mg Potassium, 5 gram of fibre, 2 gram of sugars, 10 gram of protein and then trace amounts of Vitamin-C, Vitamin B-6, magnesium, iron, copper, pantothenic acid and calcium. A good 250 gram water cooked potato serving contains less than 200 calories.

The fibre of potato has in interesting effect by binding with the bad cholesterol in our blood and help in transporting it out from the body. Together with the high supplement of potassium; potatoes helps to lower the blood pressure. In particular by its action of 'vasodilator' – to make the veins more relaxed and bigger.

Vitamin B-6 from potato plays a major role in our brain function and health by stimulating formation of serotonin, dopamine and norepinephrine.

Often potatoes are presented as glycaemic; that they spike the production of insulin. A number of nutritional studies is now indicating that potatoes are an easy form of simple carbohydrates; easy to process and absorb as energy for the body. However, when eating only potato; it does not spike the insulin production, rather just a good wave like action. After all, we do not want the pancreas to totally forget how to make insulin.

Chapter 4 - One Meal A Day.

Although this chapter is about the One Meal a Day concept – that is only valid during the weight loss program. Once you achieved your target; then go to One-Plus-Meal a Day. That is one major meal before midday and another light meal or snack in late afternoon.

As I told you before; this concept was completely out of my mind. There was no way I could ever think that I will be able to survive a day like that. Now; it is common to eat only one meal in a whole day; and maybe a snack like a soup, a slice of watermelon or veggie in late afternoon.

In all truth; this without even the slightest feeling of being hungry or craving anything whatsoever. Zero appetite for anything. Yes, I do drink around 1.2 litters of water per day.

Off course the big question you may ask, "How in the world is that possible?"

First and foremost you will need to reduce the activity of those two hormones: Insulin and Ghrelin. Ghrelin is relative easy – you just need to sleep more. Try to sleep for at least 7 hours a night and add another hour around midday. Also eat more nutritious foods, especially minerals. It might be a great advantage to take a complex mineral supplements of which Magnesium, Sodium, Potassium and some Zinc are the more important ones. Do not forget the Vitamin B-Complex in this case.

The next issue to tackle is making sure that the Insulin does not spike. Do not get a sudden burst of demand for insulin. That is easy. Just cut ALL carbohydrates and grain from your food consumption. You might be surprised to find it does not make you feel tired at all; more likely the opposite. If you can succeed in this for just a bit more than a week, you may be surprised how little you need or want to eat.

Finally; go on the Potato Only diet. For at least one week, but maybe as much as two months – eat only potato. Drink only water. Nothing else but a few 'light taste enhancers' on your potato. One effect is that you will not look forward to just-another-potato-meal; thus insulin remain sleeping. But you will also find that you eat less and less. In fact, your stomach will effectively start to shrink.

INTERESTING FACT: How big is your stomach supposed to be? The answer might surprise you. Your stomach, without stretching should be the size of your balled fist. In my case a minute 230 ml. Yip, that is correct. For an adult it should be about the size of a normal tea cup to small coffee mug. When it is full, the stomach is able to stretch – but that should be to a maximum of 40% above the rest size; about 350 ml. By that time you should feel like a bloated balloon.

So, get on the potato diet. It sits heavy in the stomach for a period between 45 and 90 minutes.

You can start off with three potato meals per day. Progressively make breakfast later and dinner earlier. Try to reach the point where your breakfast (first and main meal of day) is around 10h00 in the morning and your lighter dinner is around 16h00 (4 pm) in the afternoon. Then you are on a good track to victory.

Try to maintain this as maximum meals per day. Sometimes, if you feel good, you can skip the afternoon meal; intermitted fasting. However tempted you might feel to do so, because you are not hungry or do not have an appetite – do not skip the breakfast. You must maintain at least one solid meal per day.

One of my mistakes was not to eat anything for a day. Mostly because I did not feel hungry and I was too busy with other things. Eating the following day was sometimes a bit difficult. I urge you not to have any full-day-fasting during your potato diet days. Eat at least that once a day; preferably twice.

How long to keep up with this?

I definitely do suggest you not keep this for more than two months. Then take a break by eating more nutritious healthy foods for one month – BUT maintain your 10h00 and 16h00 two-meals-a-day routine. After that you can get back on the Potato-Only for another two month session. This will ensure your body retains its mineral, vitamin and enzyme balance.

During the break periods; DO stay away from all kinds of sugars and grains – that include milk products.

In general you can keep up with this OMAD / Potato for as long as you need. There are people that remained for more than a year on just potato diet. There are people living a good healthy life with a strict One-Single meal per day; already for a number of years. This is only your decision.

Watch your weight; watch your energy and watch your health; as in disease resistance and physical being.

You are set in the mode of One (or two) Meals A Day; and you find the Potato diet does not help you lose any more weight. Or you reach the difficult plateau of not losing weight anymore. What then?

That is the next phase of what I did. I went on the High-Fat program. That you can maintain unlimited; as long or as short as you wish. Just watch your health, energy – and the scale.

As for myself, I opted to remain on the One and Half Meals A Day, now indefinite. I feel good, energy is good, and health is good. One 'big' tasty nutrition rich meal around 10h00 in the morning followed by a light soup, vegetable smoothie or fruit mix in the afternoon. It is seldom that I will eat anything in the later part of the day or evening. Usually only when I go out with friends or family. However, the day following such a venture I am lame, my batteries are flat run out. It is like I tripped on overload. That is not a good feeling. Thus, I prefer to remain in the company, but low on the food partaking.

Chapter 5 - High Fat Diet & Ketosis.

Eat fat to lose fat.

WHAT!

Yes, you read perfectly right. A diet of high fat, lots of nice tasty foods, to lose weight. Ever heard such a controversial statement?

Yes, this is also a good general maintenance diet after your weight loss target is reached.

Let us define Ketosis first:

"Ketosis is a normal metabolic process that occurs when the body does not have enough glucose to burn for energy. When it doesn't have enough carbohydrates from food for your cells, it burns fat instead. As part of this process there is *a build-up of acids called ketones within the body."*

Let me jump back and pull an earlier statement here. *"Fat is a survival gland that protects against the starvation of sugar. It means that fat is the back-up against the depletion of sugar. Your body will not survive for longer than 72-hours without food, if you do not have a storage of fat. That is why your body stores fat."*

Thus it literally means that we need to activate an emergency state in our bodies; to force the body in start using energy from stored fat. This is not a big danger for us big and fat people, we have a lot of reserves to stand in for the body energy.

However, a state of ketosis might be life threatening for thin people. Ketosis can become dangerous when ketones build up. There are different kinds of ketones building in our blood from Acetone to beta-hydroxybutyrate and some 6 other kinds. Remember my opening statement? This book is not for those who only want to lose a few kilograms. Reaching a state of ketosis may take anything between ten days or even up to two weeks.

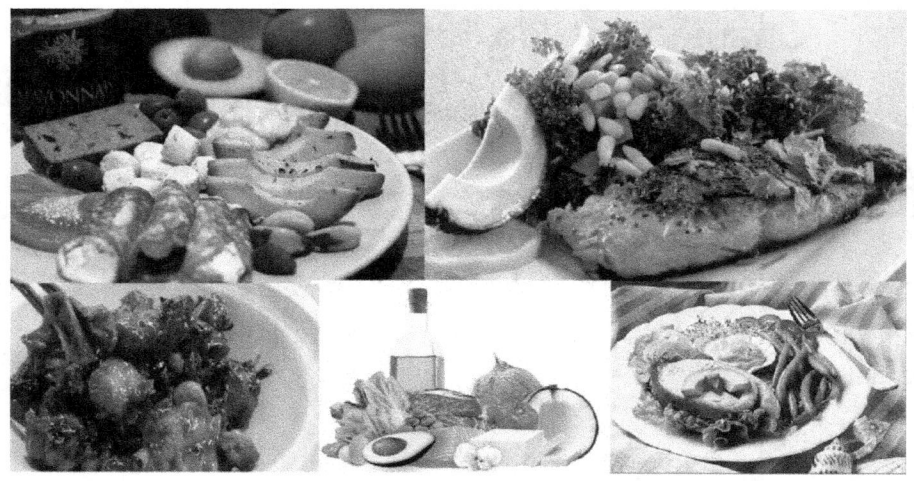

Some wonderful samples of the typical Ketogenic Diet.

The state of Ketosis can only be activated when the body is starving from carbohydrates; sugars.

Referring to that cursed word for us 'calories' - the ideal diet for balanced body weight is about 5% of the total calories to be carbohydrates; 25% protein while the rest should be 'fat'. BUT, don't jump to the butcher and buy tons of steak for three BBQ meals a day. Not yet.

WARNING: Do not go on the High Fat diet while you are doing or increasing the digestive system's pH. You do need a very acidic stomach (Hydrochloric Acid) and healthy active liver to digest the high fats.

- How to activate Ketosis?

This should be a very easy issue for yourself to determine by now.

We want our bodies to use fat as energy source (Ketosis) rather than sugar. Fat is an emergency storage. So the simple answer is "Starve our bodies from sugar." That will set the alarm bells off and all the services will be activated to run for the emergency stores.

Stop all forms of sugar.

Do not consume anything whatsoever that causes a spike in the insulin.

Sleep, relax and eat fatty foods. That will soon educate the stomach to reset for a fatty supply of food, it will send the right signals to the pancreas, liver, gallbladder, thyroid and adrenal kidneys – all will change into a Ketosis (Survival) mode.

What and how much is healthy to eat for Ketosis? Remain on smallest possible portions that makes you feel good. In my case I seldom eat any meal greater than maybe 350 ml in volume size. That is literally about a standard coffee mug of foods. Remember, fatty foods has much more energy and nutrition than sugary foods.

A nice correct term to use for searching Google and YouTube is "Ketogenic Diet." However do be selective to make sure that the article you read or watch is by people with real experience in the field or properly informed at least. There are so many fakes that jumped on the band wagon with an empty tin can as drum.

The medium chain fats does not stress the liver and gall bladder.

Coconut oil, olive oil, pasture fed beef, chickens, nuts, and some fruits like avocado are good sources.

Some fatty beef and chicken skin even bypass the liver modification.

- How do you know you have reached a state of Ketosis?

The easy and most loved answer is; "You start losing weight, quite rapidly."

When starting on the ketogenic diet, for the first week or so which we can refer to as 'transition' you will most probably find that your do not have energy. You will feel tired. Fatigue is filling your daily hours. Do not be concerned. All that is happening is that your body suddenly lacks the energy supply of sugars, it needs to kick in the emergency rescue team; and they are still sleeping. This fatigued period should not be lasting more than two weeks; then you will start to fly high. To counter the fatigue a bit, you may want to consider some electrolyte supplies. I did not, just used Himalayan salt in all my food.

You may also find the muscular system is lacking its energy and strength for a short time. This happens as the muscles are depleting their stored glycogen; and that not being replaced by the fat based energy; yet. This should not last more than a week.

At the onset stage you may find you have a bit of bad smelling breath and taste in your mouth, kind of like a tooth cavity. It is a good sign, just brush your teeth a few times more through the day and/or use mouthwash. At one time I walked with a small bottle of mouthwash in my pocket. Usually the bad breath does not stay for long, just a week or so during the transition phase.

One of the best indicators, the one I love the most. Loss of appetite. This is also part and parcel of the effect you get with the Potato Only diet. The suppression of the Hunger hormones and more active Leptin which suppress the feeling of hunger.

If you want to have solid prove, you can have a blood test done. The results should show a decrease in blood sugar levels and a great increase in ketones. Many mainstream medicals will have a fit because such could be an indicator of other problems in the body – way out of their perception of 'normal'.

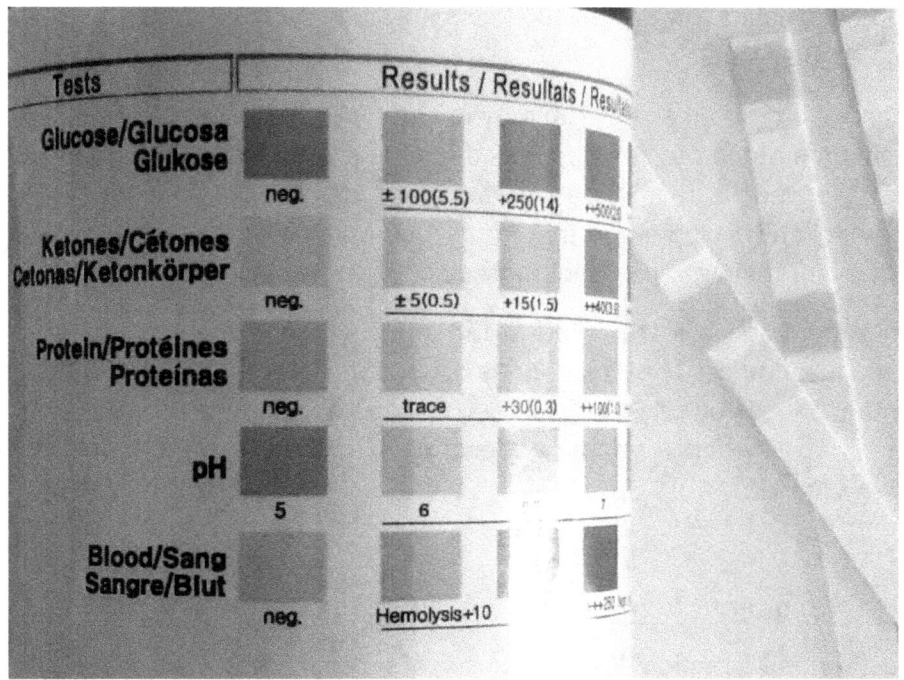

Tests	Results / Resultats / Resu|ts

Tests	Results / Resultats / Resu|ts		
Glucose/Glucosa Glukose			
neg.	± 100(5.5)	+250(14)	++500(28)
Ketones/Cétones Cetonas/Ketonkörper			
neg.	± 5(0.5)	+15(1.5)	++40(3.8)
Protein/Protéines Proteínas			
neg.	trace	+30(0.3)	++100(1.0)
pH			
5	6		7
Blood/Sang Sangre/Blut			
neg.	Hemolysis+10		++250

Ketosis testing kit, with other useful indicators.
This one was about US$ 35 and has 60 test strips.

You can also measure the presence of Acetone in your breath and urine. Breath analyzers for acetone is fairly common, for the urine you can buy measuring strips similar to those you use for measuring pH.

There is the one indicator the main stream dieticians cannot accept, yet it is fact and proven over and over. On the Ketogenic type of diet, when your body enters into ketosis state you will experience a great increase in energy and mind focus, like concentration. Ketones are a higher source of energy than sugars for the body cells and most particular for the brain. Even athletes in ketosis state reports more energy and power than when on a sugar energy level.

Then there is the digestive issues. In the beginning of the transition into the ketosis stage you most likely will suffer a bit from either diarrhea and/or constipation. When full ketosis sets in, you will have an easy and regular stool.

A final word about sleep; you may either experience some insomnia at night time but, more likely your body will require more sleep. Give in to that, the sleep is an important part of getting that fat out from your cells. All that really happens is that your body tells you to "Shut down the factory for maintenance and upgrading to a new system."

As bottom line: Weather you are in ketosis or not, there is only one issue that counts. The weight goes down. Whatever the reason, as long as that brings you back from Obese, to fat, to over weight – to NORMAL again. Then whatever name or description they might want to put on it – we are HAPPY.

- How to get out from Ketosis?

Yes, a good question. Well the answer is simple. Just do the opposite of what you did to get into the ketosis. Eat sugars.

BUT; I would suggest you do not follow that route. NEVER eat sugars, never cause an insulin spike. If you do, you will gain weight again. Rather stay on a good healthy fatty and or potato diet with some intermitted fasting in between. When you start eating larger portions of vegetables and some natural fruits; your body will quickly adopt back to using sugars (glucose) as energy source.

In fact, getting out of a ketogenic state should not take more than two days! Very easy to go up-scale again.

Chapter 6 - Problems.

- Heartburn - GERD.

GastroEsophageal Reflux Disease (GERD) is a disorder in the digestive system that affects the lower part of the esophagus. Normally, when you swallow, a band of muscle around the bottom of your esophagus (LES) relaxes to allow food and liquid to flow down into your stomach. Then the muscle tightens again when it comes into contact with the acid material in your stomach.

GERD occurs when the LES is weak or relaxes inappropriately, allowing the stomach's contents to flow up into the esophagus. This valve exclusively reacts to acid; it is not directly controlled by the brain or nervous system.

Heartburn, also called acid indigestion, is the most common symptom of GERD and usually feels like a burning chest pain beginning behind the breastbone and moving upward to the neck and throat. It feels like food is coming back into the mouth leaving an acid or bitter taste.

That burning feeling is the acid material in your esophagus; it is NOT high acid in the stomach. It is rather the opposite where low acidity in the stomach fails to cause the closure of the LES. The worst thing you can do is then to take anti-acids. Yes, it does bring a quick short term relieve; because it immediately neutralizes the acid in your esophagus; BUT it reduces the acidity in your stomach further. In longer term it makes the problem worse . . . you take more anti-acids . . . your stomach is less acidic . . . and a vicious cycle develops where the Big Pharma makes a lot of money with you only temporally feeling better but never solve the problem.

The burning, pressure, or pain of heartburn can last as long as 2 hours and is often worse after eating. Lying down or bending over can also result in heartburn. Many people obtain relief by standing upright or by taking an antacid that clears acid out of the esophagus.

The more you weigh, the more likely you are to have heartburn. Explanations vary. Poor diet, excess body fat in the abdomen, and chemicals released by body fat have all been cited as possible culprits.

I suffered from heartburn for many years, and I used thousands of packets ENO and other anti-acids. Then around 2005 I saw an article about permanently fixing heartburn by drinking the freshly squeezed juice of a lemon every morning; before eating or drinking anything else. I did that. After a month; my heartburn was gone. I could eat and drink anything; coffee, white bread, proteins, fatty foods, etc. Nothing caused heartburn anymore.

Why this is important?

Part of my weight loss program was to decrease the acidity of my stomach. That did cause a return of GERD and I had to react accordingly.

One of the major changes was position of sleeping: I had to elevate my shoulders, neck and head to a level higher than my stomach. It was not always a comfortable thing to do, but it worked fine. Also you might find sleeping on either side is less likely to cause GERD.

When I reached my target weight, and I do recommend you take a break from weight loss every six weeks, I suggest you work hard on making your stomach acidic again. This I did by drinking about 100 ml of fresh lemon juice mixed with same volume of water and a little pinch of Himalayan salt.

If you do find you have a problem swallowing food, foam reflux from your stomach and indigestion; your stomach acidity might have gone too low (pH too high). As I did make this small mistake. It is quite uncomfortable and may even cause complete emptying of stomach by vomiting.

Besides the lemon juice, a very good treatment is pure RAW Apple Cider Vinegar. Take about one spoon in the morning and another teaspoon before every meal.

In such more severe cases, you might need an external acid supplement. The only other I know of (and can recommend) is Betaine HCL. You can get various strengths of capsules; often in combination with pepsin and other enzymes.

- Thyroid Gland Issues.

This is quite an interesting point, not often considered by Main Stream Medicals. From my research I did find there is a definite link between Thyroid issues, Obese People and Stomach acidity. This is probably the least considered, yet one of the most prevalent issues.

Thyroid issues on its own are often responsible for excessive weight gains.

If you are such a case where the Thyroid might be the problem, what I explain here will definitely help you in the weight loss, regardless of the massive gain in health.

Mostly people whom are overweight due to Thyroid issues, has a general excess of weight all over the body. Heavy from head to toe, not a pot belly nor only excessive in the bums. Even a strong diet will seldom make them lose weight. If you refer to my earlier photos, yes that is the typical Thyroid problem based body.

This is the one case where genetics (DNA) could be the underlying reason or relation to oversized family members. As we are getting older this problem becomes a bigger issue and more prevalent in people.

I will try to explain on a very superficial base the intricate linking and operation of this part in our metabolic process.

You need acid in your stomach for many reasons, but one important aspect is to dissolve minerals. Most minerals are exactly the same as the elements you find on the periodic table. In other words; they are metallic based. Acid dissolves metals. Alkaline and enzymes does not.

Enabling the stomach papules to manufacture the Hydrochloric acid, your need (amongst others) Zinc, Sodium and Sulphur in your blood supply. But to get Zinc absorbed you need the active T3 hormone, to get that one you need the basic Thyroid hormone T4. To manufacture T4 your Thyroid gland needs Iodine (another metal based mineral). T4 is mostly converted into T3 by the liver, but it requires Selenium (Another metal based mineral).

For all of these, there is one critical vitamin block that you need as well. Without the Vitamin-D group, these minerals will not be available to the body as needed. You need to have some Vitamin-C in your blood and at least 20 minutes good strong sunshine per day; the body makes its own Vitamin-D. It is possible to get Vitamin-D groups in capsule supplement form. Personally I prefer the Sun.

Just to show how important this metabolic processes are for the survival of the body, there are a few glands and organs interlinking, supporting and even able to take over parts of this operations in case of failure in the Thyroid. This conversion process can in part also be supplemented by the Adrenal kidneys, liver, and even in low quantity by the Hypothalamus gland.

Now here we have a BIG problem. One which I personally also suffered for a few years and never knew how to get fixed. I had Hypothyroidism; meaning Low Active Thyroid. Periodically it will go so low that I developed goiters and other related problems.

During my pH changing of the stomach acid, everything went fine for a few months. But that is the one mistake I made – and why I keep on warning "DO NOT KEEP A HIGH pH IN STOMACH FOR MORE THAN 6 WEEKS."

For this reason, if you tend to have Thyroid issues, it is better NOT to change the stomach pH. Rather take a longer time to reduce your weight with the diet methods. Just follow what I explain on solving this issue and remain with the three diet options; potato only, OMAD and High Fat, Low Carb.

My problem was that after maintaining my stomach pH higher than 5.0 for about five months, I started developing a deficiency of minerals in my body. I realized it quickly since the most obvious noticeable was Magnesium. I started taking magnesium supplements, but they did not help.

Then I developed a goiter again, my throat was swelling up, swallowing became difficult and my voice changed. I knew immediately I had a serious deficiency of Iodine. So I added supplements of that; including the attempts to eat more sea greens. It did not help. The problem got worse.

I needed minerals in my blood; but my stomach acid was unable to dissolve them; thus my blood was unable to absorb it from my intestines. The deficiency got worse. Then, when I try to change my stomach to more acidic, the H. Pylori prevented that – AND there was probably not enough Iodine and Zinc to make stronger acid.

It took me nearly a week to find a little obscure solution to this whole dilemma. I should have realized it from my Aromatherapy education, but I think too many in-active years passed.

I bought a small bottle of Iodine solution (less than US$ 1.00) and another bottle of Magnesium dissolved in an oil base (About US$ 45). Twice every day I place three to five drops of iodine on my pulses (inside of forearm on soft skin) and rub them together. Then I spray the magnesium solution on top and rub my pulses together.

The interesting thing is that IF you have a sufficient supply of iodine in your blood, the orange/yellow stain of the iodine will remain visible on the skin for as long as two or more hours. The more quickly it is absorbed through the skin into the blood; the more deficient you are. In the beginning mine was gone in about three minutes. It is now up to about 20 minutes.

Both Iodine and Magnesium are of the few elements that can be absorbed Transdermal (through the skin) directly into the blood.

Lastly, another lessor know point. To increase the activity and operation of this whole Thyroid, T4, T3 related metabolisms; there seems to be a strong relation to the blood pH. Yes, indeed – by increasing the pH of the blood, even that little bit of 0.2 or so; greatly helps the Thyroid functions and health. To do that; the Breathing Techniques of Wim Hof we talked about earlier.

The purest, easiest solution to this whole series of problems:

Consume Vitamin-C, at least two lemon or oranges per day. Expose your skin to the sun for at least 20 minutes every day, between 10h00 and 16h00; to make Vitamin-D group. Or take Vit-D compound supplements.

Increase your mineral consumption or else supplement at least Magnesium, Calcium, Zinc, Selenium and Iodine. The best source of all of this is Sea weed and/or Sea Kelp. Alternatively is organic, grass fed chicken, beef or lamb liver. A healthy addition of organic pure mustard is a great source.

- Micro-Organisms.

Did you know that your body has more living bacteria inside it, than all the body cells together? Some researchers estimate you have as many as two bacteria for each and every body cell. However, if we add the three major micro-organisms together – the ratio is 10 for each human cell. We have more than 33-trillion human cells in our bodies.

Fungi - are microorganisms such as yeasts and molds which has membrane-bound organelles, especially the nucleus which contains the genetic material and is enclosed by the nuclear envelope. Not entirely correct, but personally I see Fungi as the plants (fauna) of micro-organisms.

Bacteria - unicellular microorganisms that have cell walls but lack organelles and an organized nucleus. Not entirely correct, but personally I see Bacteria as the insects of the micro-organism world.

Virus - an infective agent that typically consists of a nucleic acid molecule in a protein coat, is too small to be seen by light microscopy, and is able to multiply only within the living cells of a host. Viruses are even smaller than bacteria and require living hosts such as people, plants or animals to multiply. Not entirely correct, but personally I see Viruses as the parasites of micro-organisms.

Since most diseases are related to either of these three micro-organisms getting out of control ... and that is mostly due to an upset in the balance of enzymes, vitamins and minerals in your body; we need to balance the nutrients as first order in defence.

That brings us to the active duty soldiers in your body. They are called Enzymes. Enzymes are able to change molecular structures of just about anything, but they need a friendly environment to successfully operate.

Thus the simple bottom line of fighting any form of disease: Create a friendly environment for the enzymes, give them all the nutrients they require, boost the population of friendly bacteria in your body and the fungi in your digestive system.

Amongst the thousands of micro-organisms, there are two major ones which might be affected by your diet, especially if you overdo the pH in digestive system; or due to lack of minerals and enzymes. These are *Helicobacter Pylori* and *Candida (albicans)*. Since both of these are most likely already present in your system and might cause issues at any time – I consider it of great importance to include in this book.

Before I start, there is one piece of ancient wisdom I would like to share with you. This is not generally practiced in most forms of healing – and definitely not in normal allopathic medicine at all.

Do not FIGHT the invasion of damaging and bad micro-organisms. Rather PREVENT them. However, this is not always possible. When you have an invasion (overgrowth or whatever) then neither normal medicine nor herbal is very fast and perfectly effective. Here is the best advice. Fight them with bacteria.

Jip, you read that right. Rather than spend lots of energy, time and suffering on trying to fight a microbe – employ the services of a few billion microbial soldiers. All they will ask is a friendly environment and some food. You can even cultivate them outside of your body, then just send them in to do the job. The interesting thing is that bad microbes are quite defenceless against these, even if they try to mutate.

For more information you can Google "Fermented Foods" or start off with watching some videos on YouTube under "Sauerkraut" – being one of the most basic forms of how to get these killer army to work for you. The main soldiers to assist you, present in most 'Sauerkraut', are *Leuconostoc mesenteroides, Lactobacillus brevis, Pediococcus pentosaceus, Lactobacillus plantarum, lactis, and Leuconostoc fallax.*

- Helicobacter Pylori.

This chapter is important for everyone; be it for the sake of weight loss programs as presented in this book, or just normal general life. Even those who are lean or good body mass. This thing can cause big problems for every living person on Earth. The worst is the generally the medicals do not test or even consider this bacteria as a potential culprit.

Here is something you may need to know about. This is a relative new bacteria discovery – only first time isolated and identified in 1982. Since then it took nearly two decades before the real importance of this life form becomes more widely accepted. Yet, to this day in 2017, most of the older medical professionals do not accept, know nor understand this bacteria.

A shocking truth; currently about 60% of the world population is infected with *H. Pylori*. About 80% of those infected, shows no symptoms, yet. *H. Pylori* can be dormant in your system for decades, until that one day . . . As we are getting older, the acidity in our stomach naturally declines; that is often a trigger for *H. Pylori* to expand their colonization. Once the environment becomes friendly to them, they can multiply. A

Swedish research team states that both forms of *H. Pylori* causes anti-body responses and inflammation around 4 weeks after 'activation'.

Personally, looking back at my experiences; I would say that the bacteria was probably activated in late December 2016 and came to a full bloom in January. It took nearly two months from healthy to a big problem. Currently I am in the third month of self-treatment and quickly on the way to full recovery.

Next, if you go on a search about it, you will find a lot of websites and videos around the internet; many of those has no real understanding of what the hell this is. Sadly, people learn and accept wrong information. One of the good and bad opposites from the internet.

About myself; I am not a microbiologist, though it has been a great interest of mine. I am not a medical professional. But I do have a healthy mind and ability to understand. As for this microbe – it hurt me. It caused me a lot of suffering, so I made a point of studying everything I could get about it, the true, the false and the fakes. What I am going to share with you here, literally delayed the publication of this book for nearly two months – while I made war with this microbe and finally destroyed it.

Know thy enemy!

Your life or that of somebody close to you may (will) depend on it. *Helicobacter pylori* is a human pathogen associated with type B gastritis, peptic ulcer disease and gastric cancer. More commonly, the effect of this stomach bacteria will lead to bone issues, especially joints inflammation and spinal pains. But that is only the good news. If left untreated, this bacteria will eventually destroy your liver, kidneys, thyroid and even heart failure. Not to talk of brain issues!

I do not claim that the information I present here is perfect, absolute true. All I do claim is that what I have found from my research, and my own experiences – this is the best I can offer; and it is on par with scientifically proven facts to the best of my knowledge. I am sure in the coming years there will be more knowledge coming to the front about *H. Pylori*.

The problem with this microbe is . . . not enough is known about it, yet.

One may ask the question, "If this bacteria is so critical, why is there no big pharmaceutical research done about it?" The answer is quite simple. *H. Pylori* is the goose that lies the golden eggs. Literally. While this thing is running havoc in the human stomach, it causes plenty of other health problems and symptoms. Symptoms, which can easily be diagnosed and treated without killing the Golden Goose. Just think of the Anti-Acid market, big money, makes you immediately feeling wonderful without killing the cause of the acid burning. Or think about the stomach ulcers and duodenum cancers; big money for pharma and hospitals and doctors – without killing the reason why these developed.

Introduction:

Let me jump in with one of the most shocking revelations you will ever learn about *H. Pylori*. This microbe is responsible for probably more than 70% of all digestive system problems; including heartburn, GERD, acid reflux, stomach, duodenum, intestinal, colon ulcers and cancer growth, poor digestion, mineral deficiency, bad blood, tiredness, kidney problems, pancreatic problems, fatty liver, thyroid issues, and the list goes on and on and on. Probably 60% plus of digestive system related surgery would not have been necessary IF the patient or his/her doctor knew and understood *H. Pylori*.

Funny enough, not all is bad news. A 2012 study published in Scientific American provides evidence that suggests non-pathogenic strains of *H. pylori* may be beneficial, e.g., by normalizing stomach acid secretion. In addition it plays a role in regulating appetite, since its presence in the stomach results in a persistent reduction of ghrelin – the Hunger Hormone.

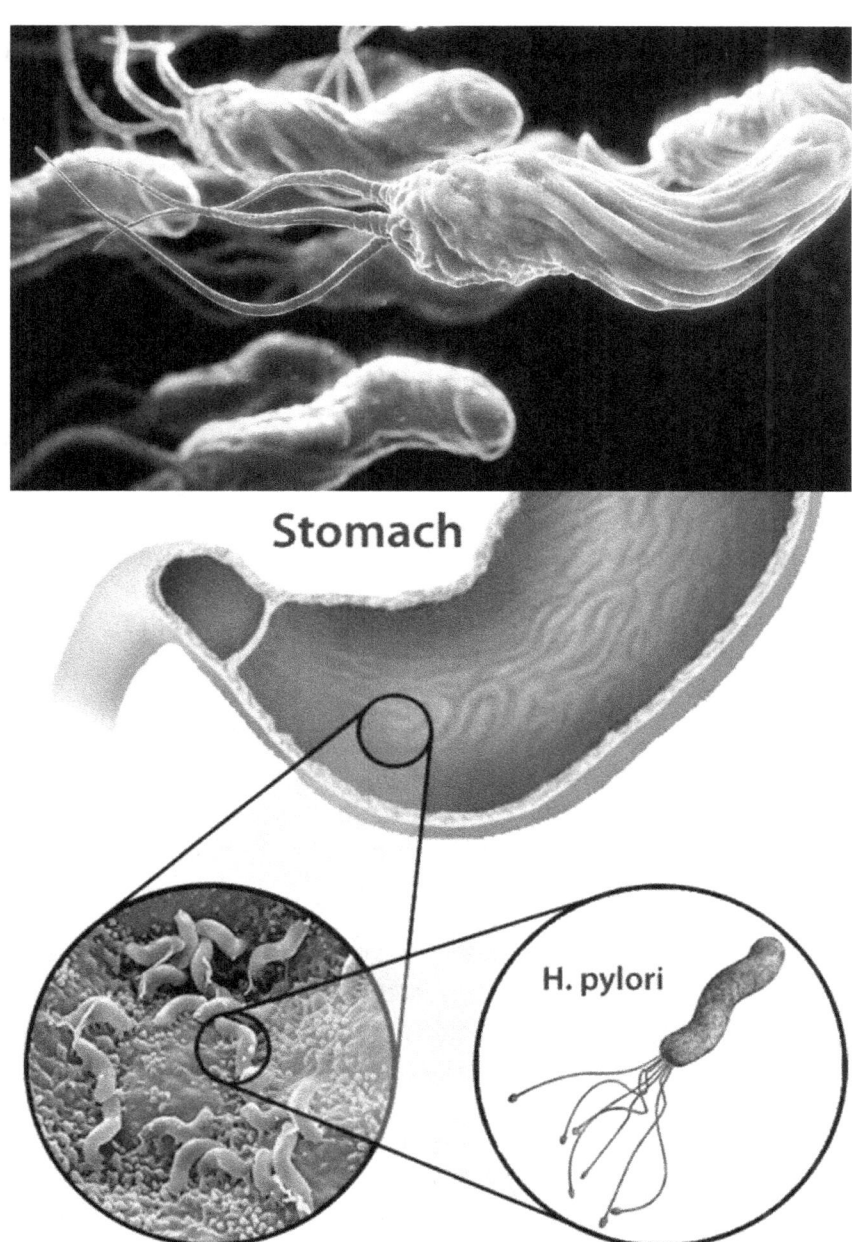

Graphic image of H. Pylori and its most favourite
colonizing region in the stomach.

Mounting evidence suggests *H. pylori* has an important role in protection from some diseases like Type 2 Diabetes, obesity and asthma. However, personally I doubt this since I definitely was obese, *H. Pylori* or not; but then I never suffered from either of the other two.

Remember what I said earlier; your stomach is the reactor of your body. Whatever happens there, affects your whole body.

Allow me to present this microbe.

The *Helicobacter Pylori* bacteria is a Gram-negative microbe that has a spiral shape. On the one end it has four to eight tentacles (called flagella). The length of this microbe is between 2 and 4 μm (Micrometre). It will take about 1,000 of these things, joined head to tail to reach a 1 millimetre length. Later procedures identified a second form of *H. Pylori* called 'coccoid', which is a curved rod shape.

The word gram-negative might have caught your attention, rightly so. Typical it is a description given to bacteria that does not stain by using violet staining methods during laboratory tests. On top of this, these bacteria has a typical double layer of membrane to protect themselves. This is one of the reasons why it is so difficult to eliminate this bacteria from your intestines. More about this later.

Although *H. pylori* was sort of known from German publications since 1875, it was first isolated in Perth, Western Australia by Barry Marshall and Robin Warren in 1982. They also proved that *H. pylori* were related to peptic ulcers. In 2005 they received the Nobel Prize in medicine for their discovery.

Just to indicate the complexity of this microbe. Its genetic makeup (DNA) was sequenced in 1989 and later more expanded. Now only three strains (of the current estimated 84 strains) are sequenced, the one (H. Pylori 26695) is known to have 1,667,867 base pairs while the other (J99) is known to have only 1,643,831 base pairs.

H. Pylori requires glucose as main energy source. Through a process called 'pyruvate' *H. pylori* is able to manufacture its own food by using lactate, L-alanine, L-serine, D-Amino acids rather than glucose or malate. It has been reported that fermentation of pyruvate produces acetate.

What exactly does this *H. Pylori* do to us?

H. Pylori can remain dormant in your stomach for decades. Often it can also be a beneficial bacteria to your system. It is only when conditions are favourable, and IF you have one of the potentially bad specimens, that they can get out of control.

This bacteria can survive in the high acidic environment (pH 1.5 to 3.5) because it shields itself with a mucus membrane against the acid environment. In addition it bores into the walls of the stomach, beyond the stomach's own mucus protection layer and there it can survive for a long time.

One miss-conception many people have is that *H. Pylori* can only survive in the acidic environment; so they drink lots of anti-acids and baking soda; believing that making the stomach alkaline will kill the bacteria. It is wrong. *H. Pylori* can successfully survive the acid because they can shield themselves. However, the ideal cultivation/colonization requires a more alkaline environment.

When it comes to calming down the burning pain of an inflamed stomach lining or ulcer, reducing the amount of acid in the stomach may seem like a good idea. But two new laboratory studies conducted by Howard Hughes Medical Institute; indicate it could be exactly the wrong thing to do.

Subjects treated with prescription drugs called Proton Pump Inhibitors which block acid production, acquired more bacteria and developed more inflammatory changes in their stomach linings.

Thus, making your stomach more alkaline may set *H. Pylori* off on a massive population explosion.

A double edge sword. In many cases, to lose weight, you need to induce higher alkalinity in your stomach. But, that may risk *H. Pylori* getting out of control. If you know for sure what to look for (in symptoms) and if you do not let the alkalinity remain for too long; then it is not really a problem to suppress the uprising of these warrior bacteria.

The stomach secretes hydrochloric acid (HCL) and mucus to protect the stomach walls from destruction. The HCL and enzymes breaks down protein into smaller peptide molecules. These enzymes require a fairly high acid environment with a pH level ranging between 1.5 and 3.5. This acid environment also helps kill bacteria, viruses, fungi and other microorganisms that enter the stomach with food.

It is now known that gastric acid decreases with age. At the Hiroshima University School of Medicine in Japan, researchers found that weak HCL in stomach of older people are the most likely reason for *H. pylori* activation. Good acid production is necessary for killing microorganisms, and poor acid production or acid neutralization with antacids contributes to overgrowth. In fact, the use of antacids can contribute to the overgrowth of many micro-organisms like; *Candida, Staphylococcus, Lactobacillus, Enterobacter, Probionibacterium – and H. Pylori.*

OK, back to the effects.

First and foremost, when the *H. Pylori* starts to multiply fast, they actually creates an alkaline environment. What happens is that they secrete an enzyme called 'Urease' which then catalyses the hydrolysis of urea into carbon dioxide and ammonia. Urease is central to *H. Pylori* metabolism and virulence, is necessary for its colonization of the stomach walls. Urease activity increases the pH of its environment; making it more suitable for *H. Pylori*.

H. pylori is the only bacterial organism in the stomach that cannot be killed by hydrochloric acid. It has adapted to survive in the stomach mucosa, and produces substances that weaken the stomach's protective mucus and make it more susceptible to the damaging effects of acid and pepsin.

H. pylori can also grow in the small intestine, sticking to epithelial cells. This adherence leads to a variety of second-messenger signals, which invoke an immunologic response against those cells causing mucosal damage by host neutrophils and other inflammatory cells.

H. pylori affects the gastric and duodenal mucous layer because this organism produces proteases that degrade the protective mucous layer. Moreover, *H. pylori* infection decreases the production of epidermal growth factor, which normally promotes healing of gastric and duodenal mucosa.

In the stomach there is an increase in pH of the mucosal lining as a result of urea hydrolysis, which prevents movement of hydrogen ions between gastric glands and gastric lumen. In addition, the high ammonia concentrations have an effect on intercellular tight junctions increasing permeability and also disrupting the gastric mucous membrane of the stomach. This can cause more havoc since the *H. Pylori* already damaged the stomach protective mucus liners.

Here is a short list of some of the most common problems caused by *H. Pylori*: stroke, atherosclerosis, insulin resistance, autoimmune diseases, heart disease, hypothyroid issues, rheumatism, gout, skin disorders, including rosacea and possibly chronic hives, some cancers, including MALT lymphoma and stomach cancer.

How does *H. Pylori* spread and infect people?

This question does not have any solid answer, yet. Some people say it originates from poorly cooked chicken, especially liver. Others say it is spread from person to person by sexual conduct or even kissing. The bottom line is purely that nobody knows. We do know one fact; *H. Pylori* is present in just about every living mammal walking on the lands of this planet.

Further, kissing is unlikely the method of transfer; unless the carrier was actually vomiting shortly before kissing! *H. Pylori* is not in the blood and it is not in the mouth. One of the reasons why it is a somewhat difficult and expensive procedure to identify. The only true, relative accurate method is by analysing stool. This bacteria is only present in some parts of the stomach, to a lessor level in the duodenum and then also quite active in the small intestines and the colon. Thus it can only be detected down from the stomach. Yes, if people are involved in some strange sexual acts, involving mouth and anus; then human to human transmission is very likely. Other than that, it is only likely to be coming into our systems via hand to mouth contamination, as in food.

Symptoms of *H. Pylori.*

Colonization with *H. pylori* is not a disease in and of itself, but a condition associated with a number of disorders of the upper gastrointestinal tract. This symptoms are not only restricted to effects from *H. Pylori*; they can be indicators of many other problems. However, if you have three or more, especially if you did have increased stomach pH levels; it is quite likely because of *H. Pylori*.

That said, the morbidly obese people (like me) have a much bigger problem to solve. If this microbe is able to help us desperate ones to lose weight, and we know we can eliminate it at the end – then so be it. Though I will say; THAT is not a healthy statement. On the other hand *H. Pylori* being a dormant bacteria and considering the extreme risks of increased heart, liver and kidney problems is a bigger problem if you do not take care. It will definitely reduce your life expectancy.

My personal view: Do not induce *H. Pylori* purposefully. But if you have it, then it is better to know that it is there and destroy it. So, even I was quite sick for a few weeks, I would tell myself to be informed and react on that.

Heartburn: Probably one of the most common symptoms. This will get worse as the acidity in the stomach is reducing. Do NOT use anti-acid. Rather use and acidic treatment like Apple Cider vinegar or lemon juice.

Ache in abdominal area: A constant ache or slight burning sensation in your upper abdominal area. Kind of difficult to pin point exact locations. In general, this dull pain will be worse when your stomach is empty. It could also be an indicator of developing ulcers in the stomach or more specifically in the duodenum.

Excessive burping: This was me. All the time, many times. The bacteria releases an excessive amount of ammonia in your stomach. Ammonia is extremely alkaline. When mixing alkaline and acid you always has a gas releasing reaction. Those gasses is what builds up in your stomach and exits as a nice long releasing burp. Keep in mind that which you ate in the hour or so since some food naturally causes gas in the stomach.

Feeling bloated: Same as with burping, only these people find it difficult to burp, thus pressure in stomach build up.

Difficulty to swallow: Food not passing into stomach. At first I thought this was some kind of intolerance for certain food. For me it started off with chicken, followed by milk. Eventually anything that is not like a soup. Steaks, corn, wheat; all omitted from my diet. It seems the food is being blocked from getting into the stomach, sitting right there at the valve. At the peak, I could not even drink water – it would just not enter my stomach. Part of this reason was the on-going chemical reaction in my stomach between alkaline *H. Pylori* and acidic HCL; it formed a lot of fine mucus like foam bubbles. Thus, lots of foam, no place for food. A very painful and uncomfortable feeling. The only way to remove the pain is to get it out from your oesophagus – vomiting. Not a nice compliment to the cook! Better cook your own food.

Nausea and/or vomiting: This only happens when the bacteria is taking over in your stomach. Because something is wrong in the stomach, the body will try to reject it and cause vomiting.

Lack of appetite: Due to the effect *H. Pylori* has on Ghrelin and also on the workings of the Pancreas (insulin) people do not develop an appetite. For us obese folks, I am not sure this is a bad symptom!

Mineral Deficiency: One of the more critical observations are when you find some mineral deficiencies. This is a critical issue. In order for the body to absorb minerals; they need to be dissolved by the hydrochloric acid in the stomach. If the acidity is weak, minerals are not dissolved and are not absorbed. Your body will eventually start showing all the signs of mineral deficiency. Especially iron, magnesium, calcium, iodine and potassium.

Anorexia: Not only the loss of weight but more critical the loss of muscle. However, you cannot be anorexic while being overweight. Your body still has lots of reserves then.

Tiredness: An unexplained feeling of being tired, exhausted or just pure feeling like jelly on a couch. This is a general symptom for anything wrong in the stomach; but if persistent over a few days you might suspect poor food digestion . . . leading all the way back to probably *H. Pylori* taking control in your stomach. In an advanced stage, this will be due to insufficient minerals and vitamins . . . again leading back to stomach pH and potential *H. Pylori*.

Unexplained weight loss or gain: Remember my advice to stop the weight loss program every two months for maybe two weeks or a month? It is not only to allow you the intake of a larger spectrum of vitamins and minerals, but also to monitor your weight loss. During those times your weight should be stable for at least two weeks – provided you are on a normal healthy diet.

Foul breath: Kind of like having a bad tooth, but it is actually methane and ammonia from the stomach and hopefully some dying *H. Pylori* bacteria. It is mostly due to fermenting foods that does not pass through to the duodenum, because the acidity is too low for the pyloric sphincter to open. This only happens when *H. Pylori* reached a controlling quantity in your stomach.

Black Stool: This one was a shock to me, I thought I had bleeding ulcers. Closer inspection I was quite baffled (before I knew about *H. Pylori*) to find it is actually a very dark green colour. This is the actual *H. Pylori* and you probably will not see it very often. What happens is that the bacteria forms a strong colony, kind of like a blob or bolus in your stomach. This can be quite painful. You will feel there is an obstruction. Then one day it will break free and either travel down the whole digestive system to exit at the anus or it may come up in a violent vomiting session. In both cases I saw the black-turn-out-to-be-green stuff. That means a lot, a hell of a lot, of *H. Pylori* being disposed by the body.

Eradication of *H. Pylori.*

There are two main reasons why eradication of *H. Pylori* seems to be so difficult. The most important reason is called 'transformation'. This is the process where DNA can migrate from one bacterial cell to another through the intervening medium. In other words, this bacteria can adapt DNA from another cell within itself or in extreme cases even from another bacteria for DNA repair. H. pylori is naturally competent for transformation and/or mutation. While many organisms are competent only under certain environmental conditions, such as starvation, *H. pylori* is competent throughout logarithmic growth.

The second is in the actual structure of the bacteria. It has two protective layers, an outer and inner. In a later booklet I will go more into the methodology of this protection and how to destroy it. For now, let us look at the various treatments.

The first I wish to present is the cheapest of all: Air. Or should I say Oxygen. In most cases with Gram-Negative bacteria, they need oxygen and in extreme cases can even manufacture their own oxygen.

However, a high dosage of oxygen is a killer for most of them, especially those that shrouds themselves in a protective layer. Oxygen literally burns them to death. Refer to the chapter about Breathing; practice that twice a day to enhance your changes of eliminating this bug.

There are many claims of this miracle cure or that miracle cure. To date, I found many a sufferer stating those are not working. Some scrupulous people makes money out of the ignorant others who suffers from a serious illness. Is it a case of the fool is easily separated from his money? Just because people are lazy to properly investigate.

I will use one maybe or maybe-not example. There is a certain company in South Africa promoting a very powerful tea. They claim this can heal your *H. Pylori* infection within 30 days, even offers a money back warranty. Obviously I was very interested. After all I am South African. So I wanted to order, but my gut keep telling me something is wrong. I set off to find out what I can, knowing some South African ethics. The product is very expensive, something like US$169 for 60 tea bags, one month of treatments. I found a few blog posts claiming this works miracles. Funny thing is that most of those blogs has just about the same posts or structure in language posts. Quite obvious that those posts were made by the same person, under different identities. Then there are a few videos of people who claim they have been healed, is not affiliated, etc. yet they promote the address details, prices and how to order just too strongly.

Here is what I found out: The tea is supposed to be a secret formulae that came through generations and has been used for hundreds of years . . . hmmm. *H. Pylori* only hit the mainstream news since the last 15 years. All ingredients are sourced from 'ALL NATURAL wild and non-GMO herbs' in South Africa (Hmmm...). The company is registered in Mauritius and the people who operate this company is a group in New Zealand. They even have a photo of them on their website. This seems to be their only product, but they have a staff of at least 20 people.

So what is in their tea? They tell us and the ingredients does reflect in the more common treatments, at very low cost. Here is the plants they claim to use: African Olive leaves, African Wormwood (Leaf & Stem), Liquorice (The Root & Leaf), Honey bush (Leaf), Rooibos tea leaves, Wild Guava (Fruit & Leaf), African Water Berry (Leaf) and Wild Garlic (Rhizome).

I do not say their tea is a fake. Most of the ingredients are well known in the traditional medicine of South Africa (White and non-white people). I am doubtful because of the company and the statements from a number of people that they did not find any relieve. One even states the tea is perfectly the same as fennel seeds! Finally, whomever tried to contact them to claim a refund or complain got absolute no replies or answers. All in all, you can get their product and try. Please let me know if you have success. As for me, US$ 169 is a steep premium to pay for something I am in doubt from day one. PS. Read their 'Disclaimer' on their own website.

Thus on to what a large number of people had success with, even if it takes longer.

Remember there are a many different mutations of this bacteria; therefore the one cure in one place might not be the cure in another location. It may kill one variety, but not another. Therefore, you will need to experiment. Also keep in mind the bacteria's own ability to protect itself. Hit it and hit it hard. That is why you read all of this so far, to understand this bacteria better.

The best results and most effective is a combination of New Zealand Manuka honey with Mastic Gum (Middle Eastern Arabian gum). The Manuka is from the wild in NZ and the bees take their nectar mostly from the very potent, famous, aromatic tree called 'NZ Tea Tree' aka *Leptospermum scoparium*. Tea Tree from the Australian outback is also a very potent plant for many health issues. That set me off on one trial, which might have made a big difference. I used the Tea Tree Essential oil (AU), five drops in 100 ml coconut oil or mixed into my natural forest honey in Thailand.

Ginger: Has been used for thousands of years as a medicinal herb. Interestingly, almost all of its claimed benefits have been validated by modern science. It helps promote healthy digestion, and is particularly helpful as an anti-nausea and vomiting remedy, from a variety of causes. Ginger has been shown to prevent ulcer formation; and it inhibits the growth of *H. pylori* in vitro.

Thyme: A popular herbal remedy in ancient Egypt, Greece and Rome, thyme was mainly used for headaches, digestive problems, respiratory illness, and as a mood-enhancer. The Israel Institute of Technology found that thyme had a significant inhibitory effect on *H. pylori*.

Fennel: Another ancient remedy for many illnesses; especially digestive system and cancer. Like many of its fellow spices, fennel contains its own unique combination of phytonutrients. Rutin, quercitin and various kaempferol glycosides gives it strong antioxidant activity.

The most fascinating phytonutrient compound in fennel, however, may be anethole. Anethole in fennel has repeatedly been shown to reduce inflammation and to help prevent the occurrence of cancer. Researchers have also proposed a biological mechanism that may explain these anti-inflammatory and anti-cancer effects. This mechanism involves the shutting down of the intercellular signalling system called 'Tumour Necrosis Factor (TNF). By shutting down this signalling process, the anethole in fennel prevents activation of a potentially strong gene-altering and inflammation-triggering molecule called NF-kappaB.

Terminalia Chebula: (haritaki in Ayurvedic Medicine) is from a tree that grows in India. The plant is used extensively in the preparation of many ayurvedic formulations for a variety of health concerns including chronic ulcers, fungal skin infections, digestive problems, constipation, heart disease, tumours, nervous disorders, asthma, and more. Its principle constituents contain chebulagic, chebulinic acid and corilagin, and its fruit is used as an antiviral, coagulant, and laxative. Terminalia also has a wide antibacterial and antifungal spectrum, and is also known as an adaptogen and hepatoprotective (liver protectant). A study at the University of Tehran tested extracts of terminalia chebula on *H. pylori*, which showed significant antibacterial activity on *H. pylori* and other bacterium.

Evodia: A seasonal tree native to China and Korea. Its reddish-brown fruit has been used for thousands of years to treat gastrointestinal disorders such as nausea, vomiting, and diarrhoea. Evodia has also been traditionally used as a painkiller to treat headaches that accompany nausea and vomiting, and relieve pain associated with abdominal hernias. Research done in Japan and Korea has found that evodia strongly inhibit the growth of *H. pylori*, which reinforces its traditional use for digestive ailments.

Liquorice: Liquorice has been used for thousands of years in Traditional Chinese Medicine as a tonic to rejuvenate the heart and spleen, and as a treatment for ulcers, cold symptoms, and skin disorders. It also has a long history throughout the world as a medicinal herb for numerous health complaints.

Modern herbalists commonly utilize liquorice in treating adrenal insufficiencies such as hypoglycaemia and Addison's disease, counteracting stress, and in purifying the liver and bloodstream. In combination with other herbs, it is recommended as a demulcent to soothe mucous membranes, and as an expectorant useful in treating flu, colds, respiratory disorders, and bronchitis.

Liquorice is commonly used in Europe to treat ulcers, and research is proving that it does, indeed, have very potent therapeutic effects. Liquorice protect the esophagus, stomach, and intestinal lining from stomach acids. In cases of heartburn, liquorice also helps repair the stomach's protective mucous lining. In the following studies, two of the standard anti-ulcer medications failed to perform as well as liquorice. Please do note; here I am not talking about the black liquorice candy we all love so much, that has less than 1% real liquorice. Please look for the root or power, it is a light brown colour and does not even taste or smell like the black sweets.

The Institute of Medical Microbiology and Virology in Germany found that liquorice produced a potent effect against most strains of H. pylori; even those that are resistant against clarithromycin, one of the antibiotics typically used in the three antibiotic treatment regimen. A study at Toho University in Japan found that liquorice are also effective against H. pylori strains that are resistant to both amoxicillin and clarithromycin, making them viable as chemo-preventive agents for peptic ulcer or gastric cancer in H. pylori infected individuals.

Curcumin: The substance that gives the spice turmeric its yellow colour. Curry powder, which is used extensively in Indian cuisine, is largely made of turmeric and other spices. Curcumin contains many powerful antioxidants and anti-inflammatory compounds, which have been shown to support colon health, a healthy cardiovascular system, and brain health. Dozens of studies have shown that it is a chemo-preventative, and more recently it has been shown to exert a strong antibacterial effect against H. pylori.

Studies carried out in the US, Italy, and Germany, produced results showing a significant in vitro effect against H. pylori, leading researchers to conclude that curcumin could be considered a valuable support in the treatment of the infection.

IMPORTANT TRUE MIRACLE TREATMENT: There is one cure, a true miracle cure. IF you can get your hands on it. But, at present it is still very expensive when you can get it. It is called Cannabis Oil (Google or YouTube 'Rick Simpson Oil'). I can't get the full thick black Cannabis oil (yet) but I do have the second best option, a bit more freely available. Natural Cold Pressed Hemp Seed Oil. The difference is that the Hemp oil is only pressed from the seeds, still powerful. The cannabis oil is distilled from the whole plant, but in particular the resinous trichomes. If the full spectrum I think it will be unbeatable. This is probably one of the reasons that Rick Simpson's treatments are so effective against most cancer types – it eliminates H. Pylori.

Are these herbs safe if you are not infected?

That's a good question. The answer is plain and easy – YES. All of these herbs can be taken both therapeutically and prophylactically. In other words, they are perfectly safe to take whether you know you have H. pylori, or whether you just want to protect yourself from its devastating effects.

Thyme, liquorice, evodia, terminalia chebula, berberine, curcumin and ginger have a long history of providing numerous health benefits without risk of side effects. And it's important to remember that H. pylori has been implicated as a culprit in several diseases, not just peptic ulcer disease. It could be residing in your liver, in which case, you could end up with cardiovascular disease or worse.

So play it safe. If you know that you have an *H. pylori* infection, take these herbs at a high dose as a therapeutic treatment for up to three months, two times a year. And if you aren't sure you have H. pylori but want to protect yourself, it's perfectly safe to take these herbs year round at a low dose.

Besides, these herbs has many other benefits for your health and weight loss.

Subscribe to my Website or Facebook. I might soon be publishing a more detailed booklet about H. Pylori. This microbe hurt me and I do not like that. I already have a massive amount of info not presented here; it will take too much space. Besides, I became quite fascinated by this Helicobacter Pylori. Certainly an interesting bacteria to study in more depth.

Keep in mind, you can effectively employ friendly bacteria like *Lactobacillus*, which you can cultivate with fermenting foods.

- Candida (*Albicans*).

I was fortunate that I did not have an overgrowth of this fungi. At least, not that I know of. However, I did find from many resources that Candida is often the cause and result of internal digestive problems with obese people. Since this fungi is present in and on just about every living human being; it is no wonder that it might cause problems when getting out of control. Getting out of control it certainly does, and very often. The correct term is 'Overgrowth'.

Candida is well known as external problem, especially vaginal for women and smelly feet and armpits for men. This is a fungi (not same as bacteria) and they like to make their palace in hot sweating damp places like the arm pits, feet and most particular in the more private areas.

It is however less known that there are more than 20 different pathogens of Candida. Less known amongst most people is that some of these Candida stuff can also survive and grow inside your various body systems. Unlike the *H. Pylori*, Candida can develop nearly anywhere in the digestive system, provided it is not too acidic. They like to occupy the small intestines and colon areas. But they can also develop into the liver, pancreas and in the urinary system; even jump the blood barriers and spread to the brain. This makes them a lot more difficult to treat in later stages.

Normally, Candida is a friendly fungi, you need them for good operations of the biological functions in your body. The problem comes when they overgrow; meaning the conditions for them are too favourable and they multiply too fast, too much. Probably the biggest problem with any form of Candida is the initial diagnosis.

Let us first take a look at this horrible (sometimes good) thing. There are two major types of Candida that creates problems for us humans. The one is *Candida Auris*; this is one people often get from hospitals. Yes, the funny thing is that the places where you are supposed to go for healing, is more often the place you might get infected. This species was only identified in 2009. Besides candidiasis, *C. auris* can cause invasion where the blood, central nervous system, liver, bones, kidneys, muscles, joints, spleen, thyroid, and/or eyes are infected. What makes it worse is that *C. auris* is increasingly multidrug resistant. The good news is that natural treatments are quite effective against *C. auris*.

Candida albicans, the better known species which affects humans, probably responsible for more than 70% of problematic human overgrowth. *C. albicans* is also a problematic infection often from hospital or other medical facilities. *C. albicans* can affect just about every organ, gland or body part in the human physics, internal and external.

In short the easy way to describe Candida symptoms is to say *"If you feel anything between slightly ill or extremely ill, you might have a Candida Overgrowth"*. Yes, that is absolutely the biggest problem. Just about any possible disease symptom (or lack of some symptoms) can indicate a Candida overgrowth.

Some of the more common indicators are: Adrenal or Chronic fatigue, Leaky gut syndrome, gas and bloating, yeast infection like a growth on skin, tongue, damp areas, irritable bowel syndrome, slow metabolism, food intolerance, bloating, bad taste and breath smell, headaches, migraine, itching skin, dry eyes, dandruff, bleeding gums, white or brownish fungal growth on tongue and inside of cheeks, sinus blockages, chronic lung infections (Bronchitis like), weight gain, foggy brain, uncontrollable muscle movements, sore muscles, mental confusion, etc.

Typical reasons for overgrowth.

Excessive consumption of alcohol, sugar and foods that easily supports growth of fungi like wheat, corn, grapes, etc. Stressed bio-system, weakened immunity system. Candida overgrowth is often caused by antibiotic medicines, inoculations as child, birth control pills, and immunity support medicines.

There are five stages or severity of Candida infection. In the initial stage one will suffer from light barely noticeable symptoms and the final fifth stage is as severe as death. In fact, many of the symptoms I presented above with *H. Pylori*; are exact synonyms with Candida overgrowth.

Candida Overgrowth Stage 1:

Affects the mucous membranes of the body, including the mouth, nose, vagina, and respiratory system. If you have five or more of these symptoms, then it is quite possible you have a Candida problem.

Symptoms include: Infant colic, childhood and adult unexplained anger/rages. Vaginal yeast infections. Severe PMS. Urinary tract infections. Body rashes. Difficulty falling or staying asleep. Eczema. Acne. Oral thrush. Allergies to foods, chemicals, dust, fungus, yeast, and/or moulds. Recurrent bouts of bronchitis, sinusitis, tonsillitis, strep, or staph infections. Gas. Bad breath and body odour. Bladder weakness. Sun or liver spots on skin. Cravings for sugar and/or alcohol. Belching. Heartburn.

Candida Overgrowth Stage 2:

Symptoms of Stage 2 includes all of stage one; plus more generalized and chronic reactions.

Unexplained weight gain or inability to keep weight on. Ear infections or tinnitus (ringing in the ears). Chronic muscle and joint pain and arthritis. Headaches. Migraine. Fatigue. Fibromyalgia. Stomach reflux (GERD). Endometriosis. Dizziness/vertigo. Bladder infection. Urinary tract infections.

Candida Overgrowth Stage 3:

At this stage, an individual's behaviour and mental health will be affected. All symptoms that belonged to stages one and two are also present during stage three, as well as:

Inability to concentrate. Serious forgetfulness. Long term and short term memory loss. Mental confusion. Not being able to think of words. Switching around words and letters when trying to speak and/or write. Loss of previous skills (such as how to type or play piano). Irrational thoughts. Unusual fears, phobias, and panic/anxiety attacks. Muscle twitching. Violence, depression, and aggression. Epileptic seizures. Infertility. Irritable Bowel Syndrome. Diabetes. Hypoglycaemia. Thyroid disorders.

Candida Overgrowth Stage 4:

Also known as "systemic yeast," this stage can result in the shut-down of some organs and systems. All the above symptoms of earlier stages will still remain in effect; but in addition some of the following:

Adrenal gland failure. Endocrine system failure. Severe constipation. Total muscle weakness. Hives

Candida Overgrowth Stage 5:

Reaching this final stage is very severe. The entire body, down to every cell, is affected. At this stage the organs shut down and the individual may go in a coma and die.

Eliminating Candida – Diet.

Fortunately, the potential treatments are also overlapping. Be it a bacteria or this fungi; there is good change that you can use similar natural treatments for either, both or none without having any adverse side effects.

Since Candida is a living organism, they need food. Therefore, if we can remove, or at least reduce, their food supply; we can starve them to death.

Typical Natural Treatments.

This is the relative easy part of Candida, provided you get into the treatment at an early stage of overgrowth. Regardless of which species is attacking your system, and regardless whether you are sure it is a Candida overgrowth or not; the natural treatment is good and healthy and will anyway benefit your weight loss program.

Guess what is very first on the list? Starvation. Since Candida just loves sugars – eliminate all sugars from your diet. Everything. Not only that grains you add to your cup of coffee, but also the sugar you find in fruits, honey, fruit juices, etc. Even things like shop bought ketchup, salad creams, mayonnaise, etc. contains lots of sugar.

Candida is a fungi, it thrives on anything that is a good base for fungi growth. Just imagine an old slice of bread covered in green stuff, or the fungi growing on a spoiled orange skin. Avoid all those kinds of food as far as possible.

Next, you fight this fungi with friendly bacteria. Those you can find in natural organic yoghurt, pro-biotic, kefir seeds, fermented coconut water, sauerkraut, etc.

Eliminate all grain products especially wheat, corn and soy.

Support and boost the liver and spleen. These are down with starchy types of food like beans, squash and bitter vegetables. Include number of teas like barley, Japanese green tea, Chinese black tea. If you can tolerate it, take a spoon full of Apple Cider vinegar before your meal.

Else, do consume some sour products like lemon and sauerkraut, which are good for the liver and heavy on supply of good bacteria.

Add bitter foods to your diet to support the intestines and colon. If you are a veggie eater, then things like kale, digestive bitters, bitter cucumber, and arugula. If, like me you have a green objection, then take the spicy road with cinnamon, turmeric, ginger, etc.

Oil of oregano, grape seed oil or extract, coconut oil, are all a strong war machine against candida.

Oh yes, did I say something about increasing the oxygen in the blood supply? Same like reducing carbon dioxide? No? Well, add in the Breathing Exercise here. More oxygen is less favourable for the majority of bacteria and fungi. It burns them because they are mostly anaerobic. High oxygen is for them like pepper spray for us; so burn them to death!

A short list of the good foods to eat, helping to get Candida under control again:

Celery, Broccoli, Olives, Cabbage, Onions, Zucchini, Garlic, Tomatoes, Cucumber, Avocado, Spinach, Kale, Eggplants, Flax seeds, Hazelnuts, Coconut oil (virgin, cold pressed), Olive oil, Flax oil, Cinnamon, Oregano, Ginger, Thyme, Black pepper, Basill, Paprika, Cloves, Dill, Sunflower seeds, Pecans, Almonds, Turkey, Chicken, Beef, Lamb, Yogurt, Chicken and Beef liver, Brazil nuts.

A final word on Candida; there are many videos and documents available on the internet, as well as support groups. All for free. In my own Facebook Page, website and YouTube channel I will also add more links and information as time goes on. See the last page of this book of link information.

Put all of this microbial problems in one basket.

I am sure you might have noticed a few similarities with the treatments, regardless the problem. Dump the sugar completely, eliminate grains, and listen to your body about food sensitivities. Add minerals, vitamins and enzymes to your food supply.

What I presented here is just a very small window to peek through. Personally I intend to write additional books about some of these problems and aspects, like *H. Pylori* and *Candida*. I just have an issue with time; and too many things to write about.

You can also find plenty of information on the internet by using Google and YouTube. See my web site for direct links to other people talking in depth about these issues.

There are three issues to keep in mind with these problems:

1. The road to health is the reverse road to disease. It takes nearly the same time to get out from a disease as what it took to get to that level. In general you can look at a period of not less than 30 days, probably around three months. Do not be in a hurry, this is not the allopathic medicine way of treating the symptom, it is about healing the body in total. It WILL take time. It is worth it.

2. Change your lifestyle to a new healthier one. Do not go back on the old bad habits, then you will suffer the same problems but much worse levels.

3. Often the problem is not where you experience the symptom. You might have a stomach issue, but it is caused by the Thyroid, which is because of a deficiency of some minerals. This is why the natural way of healing often takes so much longer than just popping a pill for a symptom. The body needs to be healed on multiple levels, over a period of time.

Chapter 7 - My Weight Loss Medicine.

Throughout this period of weight loss, I used a few herbs and spices. I am not really able to say which one or combination was the most effective. There is certainly a long list (big book possible) about all the herbs and spices that can help you, all with various contributions to weight loss, but more important is that they all are great health promoters. These are the ones on my personal list, part of my daily life. All of these items has a long list of health benefits. However, for this publication I am only going to concentrate on the weight loss and blood pressure aspects. I will list them in order of what I consider the most important or biggest contributor.

- Water.

I can't stress the importance of water enough; but all waters are not equal. To expand on this delicate yet most critical issue will take a whole book volume, thus only a very condensed bit of info here. I do intend to write a future book in this series about "Sunshine, Water and Salt".

A great part of this might be considered pseudoscience. Personally I love water and I have spent hundreds of hours studying water during these past eighteen years of my life. All water is not the same, even you may keep exactly the same molecular structure of two hydrogen atoms bonded to one oxygen atom; H2O.

Water has a memory - which I stand very firm on. Interesting development in this past two years is that scientists has found the water molecule can be programmed and it can be used to transfer information over great distances. In effect, much of the discoveries done in the field of Quantum effect has been done with water.

We know that drinking pure distilled water does not quench your thirst very well. We know that pure melted snow does not quench your thirst very well either. Whatever happened with water and whatever other material water has been in contact with – all of those does affect the water. Ever tasted the water when collecting it at the beginning of a severe thunderstorm? That water particles are so charged with positive ions; it is magnificent with wonderful feelings on your tongue. Water that comes from deep underground, then runs over stones, through forests – shade and sun, curl this way twist that way – that water is pure, extremely healthy and tastes wonderful.

On the other end of the scale, water that came from reservoirs, been chemically treated before pressure pumped for miles through steel, cement and plastic pipes to your home – that is not pure and definitely not healthy. Dead water.

Ever noticed the difference on plant when you water them with rainwater compared to tap water?

Besides all of this notes, I will probably write a book on water in the near future. Let me get back to why I place water here.

One critical aspect of losing weight is that you need to drink a LOT of water. I mean a LOT. Once your body starts consuming the fatty cells, you will have an excess of material being expelled through the liver and kidneys. Those waste material needs to be safely transported – and for that your body needs water. Another issue is that if you lose weight fast, your body will actually trim down in size. This may cause some pressure on your intestines and colon, because their space (Abdominal cavity) gets reduced. Better keep the food there more fluid.

Losing weight fast, but not drinking enough water may result in kidney problems. Especially the most painful Kidney Stones.

Water is part of the communication system in your body, just as much as the enzymes and hormones in your blood.

The water you drink should be as pure and natural as possible. This is one big problem in our modern days. Our water is so polluted, even from underground springs and mountain streams – unless you are fortunate to live in an extreme remote mountainous region.

That is where I suspect the good old lovely pink watermelon plays a very important role. The plant is filtering the water for us and it is giving life to the water.

Good healthy watermelon and good living water; a magical couple.

In general, they say you need to drink about 1 Liter of water for every 25Kg of body weight, but when you get to my old 190 Kg that would mean a whopping 8 liters a day, not something I could ever do. I will refrain by saying you need to drink at least 1.5 liters of water a day, drink more is better. AND that is of critical importance during any weight loss program.

Maintaining your health is a good natural way, the astonishing truth is that probably 30% of ALL aspects are to do with the water you drink. As I said, watch out for my next book to get a much better understanding and guidelines – to understand what importance your water is for your body.

For now, I am just going to give a basic guideline.

Drink at least 1.5 liters of water per day. That is pure crystal clear water, or maybe some tea. Not including nor consider things like juices or the water from fruits, food, soups, etc.

A good thing to consider is placing a piece of copper in at least one of your bottles water for the day. Copper is a natural anti-viral and natural anti-bacteria plus it is an element we lack in our modern diets.

Drink cold water, best is when there are little bits of ice. That water is nearly structured – electrically and magnetically polarized. Water also retains a memory, thus even it might not absorb much from the copper, but it will retains a copper induced structure. Copper promotes weight loss thought increased metabolism and especially effective against bacterial infestations. Oh, by the way of interest. Copper is essential for the body's ability to absorb ion.

Test your water to be slightly alkaline – pH between 7.0 and 7.2.

WARNING: See the chapter about pH – critically important.

- Salt.

As with the Water above, salt is also an extremely important issue, for weight loss and for general health. Not all salt is equal too. There is good healthy salt and there is bad salt. Again, this will be extensively covered in my book about Sun, Water and Salt.

The first myth and probably the worst is that you should not use salt. Cut it out. Well, there is a problem. Salt in water makes that water can conduct electricity and your body function mostly on electricity. If the salt content in your body gets too low; your whole body will face a disaster, starting in your brains and going through to every single cell in your body.

Although all of the salt we know are mostly Sodium and Chlorite, that is where the typical taste comes from – many other minerals on their own can also be as a salt-look-alike.

Forget about the 'Table Salt' and the so called 'Sea Salt' or ionized salt. Those are the worse of the worse you can wish to consume. Use that in your garden for snails or ants. That salt is only Sodium Chloride. Regardless what some foolish 'experts' claim – Nearly all common supermarket salt is primarily Sodium – 45% and Chloride 45%. The remaining 10% is moisture and a little magnesium and potassium with virtually no other trace minerals – IF any. Now, to consume sodium is very good – that is what the body uses to make many minerals it needs – BUT if there is not a good supply of magnesium; then the body can't convert the sodium. In practice you should consume Sodium and Magnesium in near equal parts. What concerns me more is the incredible pollution; especially from sea water that is dried in 'pans'.

There are four other healthier salt options that I know of. Probably more, but these are quite well known and freely available. Two of these I will not suggest you to use anymore – due to widespread sea pollution;

that is Celtic Sea Salt and Mediterranean Sea Salt. Then the two which I use from and which I consider fairly pure is foremost the Pink Himalaya Sea Salt. This is mined far back in Pakistan on the slopes of the Himalaya Mountains; and it was an ancient sea bed. Thus, literally these are ancient sea salt deposits. The pinkish salt I get and use at present is certified with none less than 82 minerals. As little as half a teaspoon a day will give you just about all the trace elements you need in your body. The other is more common in some areas, especially the far remote Sahara Desert and some parts of the Namib; it is generally called Rock Salt, though I do not have the particulars about their mineral content.

In general, the taste of all these salts are just about the same. Mostly it is the additional 'impurities' or Trace Elements that makes the one more suitable for our bodies, especially when they contain just about all the trace minerals we need. But there is another issue – The bad of table salt – where they added some additives and anti-caking agents; and often remove the trace elements for other more profitable sales.

- Watermelon.

Hmmm, watermelon as a medicine? It is sweet, juice and full of sugar? Did I misplace this thing; it should not be amongst weight loss foods! I assure you that I have done many trials about watermelon and its effects on myself over this past 9 months of losing lots of weight. When I speak to people they say I am wrong.

Initially I replaced one meal, around midday, with watermelon. No serious issue there, it was cool, refreshing and sweet energy in the hot of the day. And I lost steadily weight. Then for about two weeks I did not buy watermelon. Rather I ate some other fruits like apple, oranges, etc. My weight loss stopped after losing nearly 16 kg. Just suddenly the scale did not move down anymore. I even stop eating all other fruits, only remain with the minimum of lunch. The scale stood still for more than a week. That is it, I thought. At least I am down to 158 kg, not bad at all.

Then there was a very hot spell here in Thailand and a farmer started selling sugar baby watermelons next to the road near my home. So I bought one and enjoyed it. Generally, I cut a slice off and eat for a meal. Really enjoyable. The very next day I was 500 grams down on the scale, and my weight was down nearly every day. I did not link it to the watermelon, yet.

Then early October 2016 my weight dropped below 140 Kg. I was truly ecstatic, happy and extremely motivated. I might reach a dream weight or under 130 by my birthday in December! I stopped watermelon again. I mean, that is a sweet sugary fruit and I wanted to try lose weight a bit faster to reach my target. Two day later weight loss seized – and for nearly a week I did not lose even 100 grams. It was rock solid at 139.6 to 139.8 kg. Again I thought this was it, lower I cannot get. Just the usual happy me, content with whatever life throws at me, I am still extremely happy – considering where my weight was a few months ago.

Another few hot days and off course what is more soothing in the mouth than a nice ice cold slice of watermelon. Besides, I was very busy writing, did not want to spend much time cooking. Watermelon; love it, enjoy it. Two days later my weight started apply the negative numbers again. That was when I started to suspect watermelon has some effect on weight loss.

Come December on my birthday I was under my 130 kg target – 127.4 kg. That was also the first time I saw my one son in a few months. He was rather worried that I am sick. Same with two other friends. Even me – I do realize my weight loss is a bit fast. This time I consciously decided to experiment with the watermelon issue. I only have three kg left to go for the dream weight target of 125 Kg by end of year. Thus, I stopped the watermelon – but I changed nothing else on my eating. Lo and behold, two days later my weight stabilized and it remained steady for a week. Then I added watermelon to the daily routine again and from 20 December I lost weight. By end of year I was under my target again – a very happy 121.4 Kg.

So what is it with this watermelon? I went on a big search and believe me, there are a few claims that watermelon is diuretic (removes water from the body) but not many references to actual weight loss. Remember, losing water in your body is some weight loss but that is not the problem you really want to lose – you want to lose fat weight.

Though watermelon is sweet and wonderful tasting, it has very little in calories. Half a kilogram of watermelon has less than 100 calories. More than 90% is just water. And here I think is the secret – water and sugar; but not normal sugar. Watermelon is primarily Sucrose. It is nice smooth, cooling and filling on the stomach. But I am sure there are much more to this pink-red wonder from nature.

The best quote that says it all *"Although research on watermelon's direct effects on losing fat is scarce, the fruit makes a healthy addition to a weight loss plan."* Personally for me at this moment, it is still a mystery. It is not because watermelon makes me feel full, or replaced a meal. I did not need to replace a meal. When I eat watermelon, my weight dropped, even if such eating is in addition to my normal eating.

From my research I did find a few references to one particular mineral found in watermelons – lycopene. Lycopene is mostly found in tomato, mainly it is responsible for the reddish color in some food items. Interesting enough is that 150 grams of watermelon contains more than twice the amount of lycopene than the same mass of tomato.

Lycopene is a bright red pigment that is naturally found in the human liver, kidneys, blood, adrenal glands, lungs, prostate, colon, and skin. Many studies suggest that eating lycopene-rich foods or having high lycopene levels in the body may be linked to reduced risk of cancer, heart disease, and age-related eye disorders. IMHO, the presence of lycopene in all the organs, which are closely related to weight loss, might be a completely overlooked or at least under rated aspect of health.

Other foods that contains Lycopene, all of them associated with weigh loss programs. Tomatoes, papaya, asparagus, red cabbage, grapefruit, guava, mango, red peppers and carrots.

It seems to me that the watermelon has a trigger effect. Maybe you will find the same, maybe not. For me, when I eat watermelon, my weight drops. When I stop eating watermelon, my weight stabilizes.

- Baking Soda (Nacholite and pH).

Some people claims this is the biggest magic of all minerals. It is claimed to heal cancer, cysts, and so many hundreds of disease problems. In fact, this mineral does not really do very much in the body except it changes the pH. The correct scientific name, indicating the exact minerals, is Sodium Hydrogen Carbonate or also Sodium BiCarbonate. In common language it means there are one molecule of sodium, one Hydrogen bond and three Carbon Oxide molecules. The natural occurrence of this Sodium Bicarbonate is called Nacholite and it is abundant all over the world, wherever you find hot springs, saline lakes and volcanic waters. The natural form often contains other minerals like trona, thermonatrite, thenardite, halite, gaylussite, burkeite, northupite and borax in small quantities. To the best of my knowledge none of these are essential for the body, nor used by the body.

The big use for Baking Soda aka Nacholite is the control and or change of pH in the body. Please do refer to the full chapter about pH for more information.

- Apple Cider Vinegar.

Another item claimed by many people as the magic cure for many ailments. In fact, like with Baking Soda, Apple Cider Vinegar does not do anything in the body. Chemically and nutritionally apple cider vinegar is about 5% acetic acid with no protein, fat or vitamins and only minute traces of some other minerals. It contains for instance potassium, though a 100 ml will only have some 2% of what your body needs per day, magnesium and iron less than 1% of your requirements.

The important part is the Acetic Acid and the effect it has on the pH of your stomach. By making the stomach more acidic, it solves many health issues. Especially of you have a problem with acid reflux, GERD or H. Pylori; this is one of the better remedies.

Take about one spoon in morning before eat or drink anything else. Another topping up through the day with a teaspoon full before any meal – that is more than sufficient. IF you can get it past your taste buds. Personally, I suffer. So I rather use the somewhat less effective lemon juice.

- Turmeric.

You want to lose weight? You want to reduce high blood pressure? You want to balance the diabetic issue? This yellow root of Turmeric is one of the most powerful natural medicines you can imagine. There are many problems addressed by turmeric (and curcumin which is a main ingredient). The good effects of turmeric starts in the throat and ends at the anus; right through your whole digestive system. It is also a very powerful treatment against many bacterial and fungi issues – including H. Pylori. A very interesting effect is that turmeric also helps to protect and repair stomach walls after ulcers and bacterial damages.

Think Digestive problems – think Turmeric.

- Garlic.

A good piece of advice: Chew two to three cloves of garlic every morning, and drink a glass of lemon water after that. This will help expedite the weight loss process and improve blood circulation. I used a lot of garlic in my cooking, daily and would dare to say it was probably a good contributor to my weight loss program.

Garlic is the one addition to the cooked potato which you can make as much as you like, no restrictions. Not only will it enhance the taste of the potato; but also speeds up the reduction of weight and balancing of the digestive system.

A magical vegetable / herb / medicine. Need to clean out the blood? Think garlic. This is more effective than any expensive colon cleanser stuff (or Botox treatments) you can imagine. But garlic is much more. It is ant-bacterial, kills viruses, and many more. One can consume up to 50 large garlic houses per day without serious side effects. Well, we need to forget about the breath and sweat smell! Realistically stated, the ancient Ayurveda medicine prescribe at least five large garlic pieces per day to keep the evil diseases away from your body.

Garlic is used for many conditions related to the heart and blood system. It is used in natural treatments of high blood pressure, low blood pressure, high cholesterol, coronary heart disease, heart attack, reduced blood flow due to narrowed arteries (atherosclerosis).

Other preventative remedies of garlic is for colon cancer, rectal cancer, stomach cancer, breast cancer, prostate cancer, multiple myeloma, and lung cancer. It is also used to treat prostate cancer and bladder cancer, cystic fibrosis, diabetes, osteoarthritis, hay fever, diarrhea, yeast infection, flu, and swine flu. It is also used to prevent tick bites, as a mosquito repellant, and for preventing the common cold, and treating and preventing bacterial and fungal infections.

Effective treatments include treatment of fever, coughs, headache, stomach ache, sinus congestion, gout, joint pain, hemorrhoids, asthma, bronchitis, shortness of breath, low blood sugar, snakebites, diarrhea and bloody diarrhea, tuberculosis, bloody urine, a serious nose and throat infection called diphtheria, whooping cough, tooth sensitivity, stomach inflammation (gastritis), scalp ringworm, and a sexually transmitted disease called vaginal trichomoniasis.

Garlic is also used very effectively for treatment of abnormal cholesterol levels and stomach ulcers caused by H. pylori infection.

Think Blood issues – think Garlic.

- Ginger.

Another very powerful root to use for general health, treatments and weight loss. However, there is one controversy. Some people say ginger suppress appetite; other say it increases appetite. As for me, when I drink ginger tea I know I need to be on the lookout; it makes me feel hungry.

If you are daring, you can also go on a complete Ginger & Lemon diet; or should I say fasting. The speed of weight loss in just three days is astonishing, but you will need to fight the hungry feelings. Both ingredients have properties that promote fat and waste elimination from the body, these two together are considered to be a potent natural slimming formula.

Ginger stimulates the digestive system and is also a good treatment against bacterial infections including our big H. Pylori.

As for it's most effective properties: Think Immune system – think Ginger.

- Honey.

- It is sweet, it is sugar, it is healthy it makes fat. Sorry folks, there are two truths about honey you really need to know. It is one of the most helpful natural antibiotics anywhere on this planet. It is extremely healthy and it is the one sweet thing you can consume through any of the diet programs and health treatments mentioned in this book.

BUT: Do NOT jump overboard. Unless you are treating a condition use it sparingly. Absolute no more than a spoon full per day.

MOST CRITICAL: Your honey MUST be pure, natural 100% organically farmed, not distilled and not heated. If it taste like honey, it may not be honey. Unfortunately, when I did a honey study in 2014 I learned a stunning truth. Worldwide there is about 1.7 million tons of honey produced per year – but in large supermarkets in Europe and USA alone they sell about 4.5 million tons. The bad truth is that most of what you buy in shops are not honey at all – it is sugar blends with an artificial flavoring. They often even add pollen to make it look more authentic.

Unfortunately, it is very difficult to distinguish between real and fake. Make sure you buy from a reliable source like the farmer or bee keeper. I even insist on buying full cake at the source; easy in Thailand.

Use honey in combination with cinnamon to reduce weight. But remain with very small quantity!

- Cinnamon.

One of the big effects of cinnamon is to regulate the blood sugars and blood pressure. It has been used since medieval times to cure diarrhea, indigestion and bloating. In addition, it helps prevent the spread of cancer cells, the formation of stomach ulcers, and assists in curing bacterial infections. Cinnamon lowers blood sugar levels along with bad cholesterol levels (LDL) while having no effect on the good cholesterol (HDL). Hence, it's beneficial for both heart and type 2 diabetes patients.

Cinnamon is rich in manganese, iron, calcium and fiber. The lowering of blood sugar levels and improvement in cholesterol ratios helps to reverse insulin resistance or pre-diabetes. Since cinnamon is sweet to the taste, it also satisfies the craving for sweet foods that generally afflicts diabetics.

A teaspoon of cinnamon a day will definitely increase your weight loss. You can use cinnamon with the potato diet, effectively. At the same time it reduces blood pressure, risk of heart disease – and it helps to eliminate bacteria.

Cinnamon helps prevent this increased storage of fat and enables you to lose weight. It influences the manner in which sugar is metabolized by the body and prevents the transformation of the metabolized sugar into fat. Cinnamon delays the passing of food from the stomach into the intestine. Hence, you feel satisfied for a longer time and eat less. This also helps you lose weight and changing to the One or Two meals a day program.

I prefer to use cinnamon together with either honey or lemon juice. Amazing cooking couple and for smoothies. Do not use too much cinnamon, a teaspoon per day is about the upper limits. If you use more, cinnamon may spike your insulin secretion.

A personal note: I found H. Pylori is defiantly not happy when I eat cinnamon, they pull out all their armies when cinnamon landed in my stomach. Cinnamon is known to kill them!

- Black Pepper.

There is a suspicion that piperine (a component of black pepper) might be an assistance in any weight loss program. However, I cannot find another peer review or verification of this yet. All I do know is that you can use black pepper in your cooking, as seasoning as much as you like. It does not spike the insulin.

Besides this, black pepper is considered a medical spice in Asia where it is applied in cancer treatments, improves digestive action in stomach, is anti-bacterial. The main benefit, in my humble opinion, is that Black Pepper promotes the dissolving and absorption of minerals form the intestines into the blood.

Use pepper and fermented pepper (Worchester sauce) instead of Italian kind of oily dressing for your food.

- Mustard.

Seeds and leaves of the mustard plant are rich source of minerals such as selenium, calcium, magnesium, phosphorous, iron and potassium. It is also a good source of dietary folate, vitamin A and a number of trace elements needed in our bodies, like copper and zinc.

As with black pepper, mustard in itself will not be of much assistance to losing weight. But, it is a nice addition to your food as flavoring. Although, there are those that states it is a good addition to speeding up weight loss because of the high Vitamin-B complex content. Personally I would subscribe to that notion, I think it helps to break some of the plateau that we can land on during the program, especially when on high fat diet.

Mustard has been used for a long time, and proven itself in the treatments of: Gastrointestinal cancers, asthma, rheumatism, arthritis, joint, and general muscular pains. And then there is the one thing where mustard excels: breaking down of the bad cholesterol in arteries and veins; this is mostly due to the high levels of niacin in mustard seeds.

Mustard has been used in the Middle East for centuries to fight viral and bacterial attacks. The large blend of minerals present is a great fortress to assist your body with defenses against diseases.

- Chili Pepper.

Remember when I talked about the depletion of Vitamin-C when fruit is harvested? There is one little understood issue: Most Red Chilies has this funny thing that it not only contain about seven times more vitamin-C than an orange (per weight measure) – but it locks the Vitamin-C potency for a longer period of time.

Chilies are a good source of vitamins A, B, C and E, beta-carotene, folic acid and potassium; it also contains the minerals molybdenum, manganese, folate, potassium, thiamin, and copper.

Off course we want to know about the weight loss values. Well, Chilies is the napalm of spices for weight loss. It will kick start any lazy fat searching hormone in your body. Some studies shows that you can increase the weight loss temp by as much as tenfold, just by adding a healthy pinch of hot chili to your meal. The action is a very basic one; Chilies increase fat burning by oxidizing the layers of fats in the cells. In addition to this, the main component in hot chilies (the thing that burns your tongue) is capsaicin. Studies in Australia found that capsaicin promotes the loss of weight by reducing appetite, activate the 'feel full' hormone Ghrelin and reduces the activities of insulin.

My advice; do not keep a salt pot on your dinner table; keep a pit of hot dried chilies. Oh yes, suffer from heartburn. Like I used to? Well, then you first need to take care of that – use Apple Cider and/or lemon juice to get it sorted out. I could never ever eat hot spicy food anytime in this past 25 years. Now, I almost cannot eat if there is no spicy chili in my food!

NOTE: By no means is this a full list, it is what I have, what I used and still use in my cooking and foods. Just to describe some of the lessor know issues about our spice racks and food. There is a myriad of information available all over the internet. Just be careful what you believe, always verify it from at least three different not related sources.

Chapter 8 - An Open Letter to myself.

A question people may ask by now is "What exactly did you do and what do you suggest". Well, I can't give you any such advice. After all, I am not your medical doctor! But hypothetically let us say I have the magical opportunity to talk to myself a few years ago. Something like a time travel. Or better, through the magic of time shifts I can send my younger self a letter – What would I tell Corrie to do? Let us say I could send this back ten years.

Hi Corrie,

This is the much more experienced and bit older yourself sending you this very interesting letter. Yes, I know it sounds strange, but true. See, I am now living in 2017, to be exact it is April 2017. I want to tell you about some of the most amazing experiences I had and give you some very important advice. Please do read this letter carefully and get on your computer, research this information.

Hey man, it is time to get off your fat arse and start losing weight. Yes, I am talking straight to you. If you go on with this fat body of yours you are going to get lung cancer and suffer a lot. After that you will barely be able to walk. Your weight is going to be around 200 kg. Just think of your poor sons who might need to rent a crane for moving your dead body around at your funeral. You are too heavy for them to carry.

But don't worry myself, I will tell you exactly what I did and a few things that you will need to change. Hey man, I am now 98 kg of weight. Can you believe that! My clothes are down to a size 40 on trousers and LL on shirts. Sitting in a bus or airplane is a pure pleasure, and nobody suffers around me anymore. I have lots of energy, kind of like that time when we were only 20 years old.

OK, I am limited on paper size. They only allow me two pages plus another three pages added as guidelines. Let's get on with what I need you to do.

First and foremost; you must immediately stop eating any sugars. I really mean everything that is sugar, contains sugar, even fruits and coffee. The same with grain products. Take that microwave in my office and throw it out the window. You need to learn cooking more food yourself, on infrared heat. Tell you, there is an amazing variety you will learn about cooking. Use the internet, plenty of wonderful recipes.

Oh by the way; I am not going to tell you to do lots of exercises. I know you hate it, but believe me now I am doing quite a bit and I enjoy it. Just do some movements, swinging arms and legs and walking. Just to get your poor body mobile and balanced again.

For every aspect of this program, there is one page allowed which I will add on to the end of this letter.

The next thing you are going to start doing, right after reading here is a series of Breathing Exercises. It is not strenuous, but extremely beneficial. Can you imagine; I can now hold my breath for a bit more than five full minutes. Yip, that is right. This only takes 15 minutes per cycle – do at least twice per day.

Clean out your fridges at home and in the office. Only stock up with water . . . and potatoes. Yes, you are going on a potato only diet. Lovely? I know you think it is fun, you like it anyway. It sounds like fun, but in truth it is a bit difficult. The reason why you will do that is to get off the system of eating three times per day, plus snacks. It will also help you to get your body away from that crazy hunger feelings and in particular the want for sugar. For the next two months (60 days) you can eat only potato, as much as you want but preferably only boiled in water. Yea, Ok man. You can use some other things, but refer to the page about this diet. In the first two months you can expect to lose up to 20 Kg. Yes, are you not listening – I said 20 KILOGRAMS. Get on it, start right now.

And by the way, keep record this time. Take photos at least once a week of you on the scale. Don't be as stupid as me. Why? Because you are going to write a book about this to help other people like us. By the way, do you know what they call us? Mortally Obese. Yip, on the way to death, fast track.

Oh yes, sorry I forgot something. Try to eat your breakfast later every day. Best time to go is for eating first time around 10h00 in the morning. Dinner is gone, lunch is late in afternoon around 16h00. Eat or drink absolute nothing else at any time except water. Oh, don't worry. You will get so tired of potato only; you will not even want to face the cooking of it anymore. Eating less times and less potatoes will just become a normal issue on daily basis.

After this first two month session, you get off the potato and eat normally. Not any crap. Please do remain with two meals a day and remain with healthy nutritious foods. Think of raw salads, mostly.

When you start the next session, I want you to slowly increase the pH of your stomach with baking soda; but PLEASE do not let it go higher than pH 4.0. You have a bacteria in your stomach and that thing might get out of control, causing a lot of discomfort. Yes, you heard me right. You have a bug in there that is potentially dangerous. I include a chapter here for you with much of the details, how it works, what it does and how to get it out of your system. That is a very important issue you have to take care of. Please. That thing is called Helicobacter Pylori or in short H. Pylori. Please do more research about it and how to eradicate it. It is not so difficult. While on this trend, also review your knowledge of Candida again, that is not your problem but of a close friend.

Ok, when you start your potato diet again, remain on the two meals a day, for now. You will continue to lose a few more kilograms. Then it will flat out and you will find it very difficult to get it further down. It is called a plateau. That is when you will change over to a lovely diet.

That new one is the High Fat, Low Carbohydrate. In fact the carbohydrates should not be a problem since you have already eliminated that from you food list. All you need to do now is to change your potatoes over to fatty foods.

Yes, wipe that dumb look from your face. I say you can eat some steaks, bacon, butter, avocados, nuts, etc. After being on potato only for few months, I would think you will be happy! This fatty kind of diet will cause an effect called Ketosis in your body. Go Google that for more info. Don't worry, you have LOTS of storage left to keep your poor body running on empty; using only the stored fats for quite a long time.

An important thing to keep in mind. Do not make the same mistakes I made. Only run the mono-type diets for up to two months, then take two weeks or up to one month off by eating all sorts of other healthy, nutritious foods. That is mostly to keep your systems in good operational order and to restock on minerals in your body.

Remember, keep a nice record of everything you experience, you will write a book about all of this by the time you have lost a fabulous 90 Kg of excess weight.

Take care my dear self, I hope you will have a long life; as I expect for myself now.

Your 98 kg self,

5 April 2017.

Chapter 9 - Staying slim and healthy.

Once you understand the basics of what I wrote in this book above; and you know how to successfully lose weight with the Potato diet alone, you have the basics experience of controlling stomach, intestinal, urine and blood pH – and finally the bit of info I presented about the Ketogenic diet – THEN you should never experience any difficulty to maintain your weight.

However, there will always be a few small rules.

Remember; you cannot run your body energy on both Glucose and Fatty acids. You will have to pick either or. Considering all the benefits, I personally rather opt for the tastier, slower burning more enjoyable energy sustaining fatty acids – Ketogenic diet.

Stay as far away as you can possibly be form ALL kinds of sugar. Even limiting your consumption of fruits and vegetables that does contain good healthy glucose. Every sweet bite you take, will spike your insulin – and will cause many issues in your body. In my personal case; if I now eat something sweet it literally makes me nauseas; thus I better leave it alone. Even now I do not have a weight problem anymore, I still find I have absolute no desire or craving for any sweet thing.

Grain products is another whole line you should try to keep away from your body. It Is not as serious as the sugar issue; but always keep in mind the GMO, mass agriculture practices with all sorts of chemicals . . . I think better let it be. Though I do admit, maybe a rye bread roll in a week is acceptable for me, especially to make a hamburger.

Even calves do not drink the milk form their mother after some two years. Remain a distant form most dairy products – unless you use dairy to cultivate Super Foods like fermentation, etc. Even then, try to ensure your products are from organic, natural grass fed animals.

Chapter 10 - Additional Information.

NOTE: As a general rule of the thumb, an issue to keep in your mind. Minerals are elements, and mostly a form of metal. Therefore they are usually heat tolerant. Cooking food does not destroy the value of minerals. On the other hand, most vitamins are not heat tolerant – thus when you heat food (like pasteurization) or cooking you will most likely destroy or reduce the value of the vitamins. Many of the natural vitamins does not store well either. Enzymes and microbes are always destroyed when heated. Thus a great cooked cabbage will not make a good sauerkraut. Pasteurized, canned and dried foods are mostly depleted of their nutritional values – except for minerals.

- Notes about Vitamins.

There are various groups of vitamins, each with their own unique properties; usually identified by an Alphabet character and a number. Basically vitamins are organic in nature and essential nutrients to be included in your food. There are some vitamins that are made within the body, but these usually requires another vitamin as raw material. There are 13 vitamin groups that your body needs for proper function. They are vitamins A, C, D, E, K and the Vit-B complex (thiamine, riboflavin, niacin, pantothenic acid, biotin, vitamin B-6, vitamin B-12 and folate).

Vitamins are important for metabolic, biological and other processes in the body like metabolism and gland functions. Gland functions includes your body's defence against diseases. It is not a source of energy for the body and it does not serve as a building block for cells. Although vitamins are not generating energy, they are essential for the body to generate energy from other material, we can actually say Vitamins are a Catalyst for the body.

Vitamins are not stable substances, and are susceptible to destruction by heat, light, water, radiation or changes in acidity.

Vitamin-A is the group of unsaturated organic fat soluble compounds that promotes growth. This vitamin becomes increasingly more important for the immune system as we get older. High vitamin-A foods include sweet potatoes, carrots, dark leafy greens, winter squashes, lettuce, apricots, cantaloupe, bell peppers, fish, liver, and yellow tropical fruits like mango, papaya, etc. Consuming Beta-Carotene, also allows the body to manufacture its own Vitamin-A as required. My primary source is carrot and yellow tropical fruits, in particular papaya and mango.

Vitamin-B is water soluble vitamins that plays a major role in cell metabolism. There are eight Vitamin-B's and a combination of them are usually referred to as Vitamin-B Complex. These water soluble vitamins are easily storable. Although we do need and should maintain a good intake of the whole Vit-B group, we should make sure of plenty B1, B2, B3, B5 and B12. If you do have a diabetic problem, then Vit-B1 is critically important. For the purpose of this program I used the good old Marmite as my major Vitamin-B complex source; a small teaspoon serving size contains nearly all the Vit-B group you need, including B12.

Vitamin-C is best known for its boosting of the immune system. It is a water soluble vitamin; and it is not stored in your body. In truth most of what people think they are taking in as Vitamin-C is not Vitamin-C anymore. In general the fruits you consume starts losing their Vitamin-C vitality within the first few hours after being harvested. Vitamin-C is especially unstable and degrade through heat, oxidation and even exposure to oxygen or in alkaline conditions. Storage also destroys vitamin-C. Progressively over a day or so all the value and potency of Vitamin-C is depleted. Heat and sunshine speeds this loss process up.

Vitamin-C is needed for the synthesis of collagen, a protein that helps with wound healing. An important factor to keep in mind if you had an H. Pyloric infection. Vitamin-C also decrease your risk of chronic diseases such as cancer and heart disease. Vitamin-C is the basic requirement for the body to manufacture Vitamin-D.

Read again: Vitamin-C cannot be stored. It cannot come in a supplement or pill form. The only good source is very fresh from the farm fruits. Low levels of Vitamin-C in our bodies tends to increase the risk of fat storage. In other words around: If you have high levels of Vitamin-C; it is easier for the body to extract the fat from storage for energy.

On average we need about 90 mg of Vitamin-C per day.

Vitamin-D is a group of fat-soluble vitamins and they are important for intestinal absorption of major minerals like Calcium, Iron, Magnesium, Phosphate and Zinc. I do not know which foods you can eat with high levels of Vitamin-D. In the natural condition your body manufactures its own required Vitamin-D group by sunlight. The raw base material required is Vitamin-C, then exposure to sunlight. On average where I am about 20 degrees from the equator and full strong sunlight – I need to be exposing as much as possible skin to the sun for at least 20 minutes per day. Vitamin-D is stored in the body cells and will remain ready when called upon for up to three days. My diet is very heavy in the minerals Calcium and Phosphate, adequate Vitamin-D is required since this controls the blood levels of these minerals. A shortage of Vitamin-D will affect your bone structures, brain activity and also might be playing a role in diabetic conditions.

For my program, I eat at least one citrus fruit in the morning, or more often the juice of up to three fruits; at least an hour before I go work in the garden for at least one hour daily, full sun dressed only in a short. I am not yet sure if this is one of the main contributing factors (I suspect it) but I used to suffer from lots of leg cramps. I did not have any leg cramp for many months now.

Vitamin-E & F. One of the vitamins I do not really consider important, although it is suspected to be helping against arteriosclerosis by cholesterol. This vitamin is high in certain grain oils like Soy, sunflower, wheat germ, etc. It is also present in most legumes and nuts, thus whatever minute quantity your body needs; it is already present in just about any food you might eat.

As for all the rest of the vitamins, I do not consider any of them important for this exercise. Besides, the body requirements of these are such small quantity – and whatever is needed will be in most foods that is also supply Vitamin A to C.

- Notes about (Nutritional) Minerals.

Some people says there are 84 elements which are required for the healthy human body. In truth the number is a much easier 19 elements and 4 gases. However, we do find other minerals which are actually two or more elements that combined i.e. Sodium & Chlorine which forms Table Salt. Most of these are only trace minerals, meaning they are is such low levels it is not even present in every drop of blood. But, there are a few minerals that are important to us – and for our weight loss, these are very important. The minerals we really do need in larger quantity is called Macro Minerals and those that are only in minute quantities are Trace Minerals. In general minerals are exactly the same as most Chemical Elements, as in the Elementary Table.

Calcium. The first of the critical important minerals for our bodies. It binds very easy with a number of other elements. Most important for us is the formation of bones, teeth, nails and hair. Calcium regulates blood pressure and prevents insulin resistance. In addition to this, Calcium is often used by the body as base mineral to make its own biological Sodium which in turn is of critical important to our electrical body functions, nervous system and brain. Most dietary Calcium is from dairy products, however, there are now reasons to believe that source is not really healthy for humans anymore. The other main supplies are from certain seaweeds, nuts like almonds, hazel, pistachio, molasses, legumes (beans), soy beans and milk, some fruits like figs, oranges, vegetables like broccoli, rutabaga, kale and okra.

On average we need to consume about 1 gram of calcium per day. In weight mass about equal to a regular paper clip.

Phosphorus. This works with the Calcium to strengthen our bone structures. Phosphor / Phosphates are also a very important part of each cell in the body's membrane and plays a vital role in energy production for your body. If you have a high level of Phosphor, the body absorbs less Calcium and if high level of Calcium it absorbs less Phosphor – the two goes together and the body try to maintain them in perfect balance. To generate and absorb sufficient Phosphor, you need a good level of Vitamin-D. Phosphor is quite important in detoxify your body on the one hand and the other in absorbing nutrients and effectively utilize it for energy.

For this weight loss action an adequate supply of Phosphate is quite important since it is the most active mineral to control the pH level of the body cells. When terminating the weight loss phase, phosphor becomes very important to rebalance the stomach and intestines. Time to take additional supplements; but remember Phosphor + Calcium + Vitamin-C + Sunshine all must go together.

My preferred foods for Phosphor is Sunflower seeds, white beans, Tuna and potatoes. Other good sources are Broccoli, beef and dairy products.

On average we need to consume about 0.7 gram of Phosphor per day.

Potassium. An important substance for electrolyte that conducts electric charges throughout your body along with sodium, chloride, calcium, and magnesium. Potassium is crucial to heart function and plays a key role in skeletal and smooth muscle contraction, making it important for normal digestive and muscular function. Any actions involving the heart, think Potassium since it has proved that higher intake of Potassium reduces risks of stroke and other heart diseases.

Overweight people, especially the obese, always has a hand-in-hand condition - High blood pressure. Potassium is the one mineral that enables and promotes reduction in blood pressure. The other common problem for big people is diabetes; and here again Potassium is effective in normalizing blood sugar.

Foods that are high in Potassium: Potatoes, Avocado, Cantaloupe, baby carrots and banana. There are many other foods as well, but not so high levels.

On average we need to consume more than 4.5 gram of Potassium per day. Few people get sufficient volume from a normal diet.

Sodium. Think table salt - Love it, Hate it. "Cut it out' they say. In truth you can't, no sodium and you will die quietly. But they are also right, we are usually overdosed on sodium. These days it is not only the salt you spread over your meal, but it is in nearly all foods you buy, often you are not even aware of it. For instance, did you know the famous Coca-Cola not only contains a large amount of fructose – but also up to 75 mg Sodium Chloride?

Sodium is important for your muscular functions, blood compounds and brain actions. Any and every little electrical impulse throughout your body requires sodium. Other basic functions include; Eliminates Excess Carbon Dioxide, Regulates Glucose Absorption, Maintains Acid/Base Balance Regulation of Fluids (One of the most notable effects is the ability to balance the osmotic pressure in the human body's cells), Balance of Ions, Maintains Heart Health. Sodium plays a vital role in maintaining the blood pressure of the human body, but an excessive increase in its content can dramatically boost the blood pressure and result in serious health complications.

Normal table salt is a combination of Sodium and Chloride; about 50/50 ratio. Some other forms of salt like Himalayan has additional trace elements which makes it healthier to the human. Just about every single type of food we can imagine to eat, contains sodium.

Suitable dosage of sodium is around 1.5 grams per day. Since most food salt is about 40% of sodium; you should consume between 1/3 and 1/2 a teaspoon per day, in total.

Magnesium. Magnesium is a mineral used by every muscle and organ in your body, especially your heart and kidneys. Most magnesium is stored in your bones and organs, where it is used for many biological functions. Yet, it's quite possible to be deficient and not knowing it, which is why magnesium deficiency has been dubbed the "invisible deficiency." Symptoms could be unexplained fatigue or weakness, abnormal heart rhythms, muscle spasms and even eye twitches.

Later findings indicate that the importance of Magnesium has been greatly understated in recent times. Now researchers find there are more than 3,700 bindings and activities in the human body that requires magnesium. Primarily the actions are divided into five groups: Activating muscles and nerves, creating energy in your body, helping digest proteins, carbohydrates, and fats, serves as a building block for RNA / DNA, precursor for neurotransmitters like serotonin.

A lack of Magnesium can result in many different diseases – physically and mentally: Anxiety, panic attacks, diabetes, migraine, nerve, muscle and skeleton problems, osteoporosis, rheumatism, PMS difficulties, tooth decay, insomnia, etc.

As if a shortage of magnesium is not critical enough; if magnesium is out of balance with Calcium, Vitamin K2, Vitamin-D – and others, those does not perform their duties either.

It is an amazing fact that the majority of Western people are deficient in magnesium. One of the better indicators are your bowl movements. If you have a constipation problem, then you probably lack magnesium.

The best way to increase magnesium consumption is by juicing a mixture of green vegetables and herbs. Besides this, there is not much to do other than supplements. The main reason is that modern agriculture has basically depleted the soil of magnesium elements to the plants, thus our foods does not contain much of these anymore.

Supplements are also a bit complicated since magnesium is not available nor to be consumed in 100% pure format. Thus we need to look for combinations, the following are my preferred compounds: 60% Magnesium Oxide, Magnesium Citrate, Magnesium threonate.

Our bodies need about 0.4 gram of Magnesium per day.

Sulphur. Sulphur/Sulphate is also a component that we usually have in abundance. Sulphur is a very important mineral to consume and have in our bodies; in fact, it is the third highest by volume and important elements (after Calcium and Phosphorous).

There is often a misconception that MSM is a not-to-consume chemical, mostly used in food preservation. MSM (Methylsulfonylmethane) is the organic form of Sulphur, as your own body requires and uses it. The most obvious symptoms of low MSM is chronic fatigue, depression, high physical sensitivity to stress and a myriad of other degenerative diseases. Sulphur in balanced volume, is a preventer of cancer, good detoxification, prevention of the bad intestinal parasites and worms, fighting autoimmune disease and prevention of diabetic conditions. MSM is a critical component to reduce inflammation.

Good sources for sulphur is garlic, onion, beans, kale, organic eggs, and Brussels sprouts.

Our bodies need about 1.5 up to 3 grams of sulphur (MSM) per day.

Chlorine. It is also the other 50% in most table salts – Sodium Chlorite. (Chlorine being Chlorite).

Trace Elements. Never think that because these elements are only required in extreme low levels for us human bodies that they are not important. As I have explained earlier you truly need some of them, even a tenth of a drop spread through your blood might be all that is required. Yet, if you do not have that minute quantity – you risk developing serious issues. A good example of this is the very common problem of Low Thyroid issues.

- The Periodic Table of Elements.

This is just a special section for the real curious; listing all the elements we know that are important for human existence and health. All of these are used in or by our bodies to form, maintain, repair and preserve our physical living being.

Basic Critical: Hydrogen, Carbon, Nitrogen and Oxygen.

Very important, large quantity: Sodium, Magnesium, Phosphorus, Sulphur, Chlorine, Potassium and Calcium.

Essential Trace Elements: Vanadium, Chromium, Manganese, Iron, Cobalt, Nickel, Copper, Zinc, Arsenic, Selenium, Molybdenum and Iodine.

Found but functions not clear: Aluminium, Germanium, Bromine, Rubidium, Strontium, Cadmium, Tin and Lead. These might all be contaminants rather than useful, mostly heavy metals that is not easily disposed of by the body.

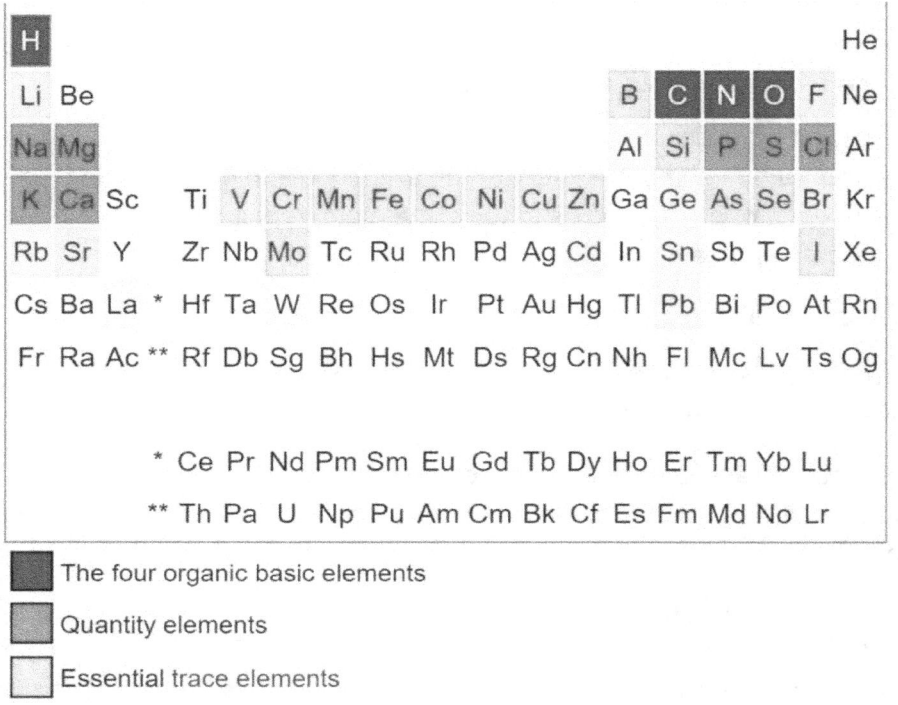

H																	He
Li	Be											B	C	N	O	F	Ne
Na	Mg											Al	Si	P	S	Cl	Ar
K	Ca	Sc	Ti	V	Cr	Mn	Fe	Co	Ni	Cu	Zn	Ga	Ge	As	Se	Br	Kr
Rb	Sr	Y	Zr	Nb	Mo	Tc	Ru	Rh	Pd	Ag	Cd	In	Sn	Sb	Te	I	Xe
Cs	Ba	La *	Hf	Ta	W	Re	Os	Ir	Pt	Au	Hg	Tl	Pb	Bi	Po	At	Rn
Fr	Ra	Ac **	Rf	Db	Sg	Bh	Hs	Mt	Ds	Rg	Cn	Nh	Fl	Mc	Lv	Ts	Og

* Ce Pr Nd Pm Sm Eu Gd Tb Dy Ho Er Tm Yb Lu

** Th Pa U Np Pu Am Cm Bk Cf Es Fm Md No Lr

■ The four organic basic elements

■ Quantity elements

□ Essential trace elements

- How long does the food stay in your body? (*Thank you Emma*).

In the stomach, food tends to hang around in the stomach for different time scales depending on a variety of factors including the amount of food you have consumed, how much fat it contains, and also the acidity of the stomach. Here is a more detailed breakdown of food types and the average time it will remain within the average healthy person.

On an empty stomach, water will pass through to the intestines within minutes.

Fruit juices will take around 20 minutes.

Light fruits like watermelon, cantaloupe around 30 minutes.

Fish - cod, scrod, flounder, sole seafood - 30 minutes.

Heavier fruits like oranges, peaches, and avocado - 45 minutes.

Fish - salmon, salmon trout, herring, (more fatty fish) - 45 minutes.

Vegetable salad or cooked - 45 minutes.

Carbohydrates & Starches like corn, potatoes, squash, and rice – about 1 hour.

Grains like brown rice, cornmeal, and oats - about 90 minutes.

Legumes like beans, chick peas, peas, etc. - about 90 minutes.

Seeds, Light nuts and Soy beans - 2 hours.

Poultry meat like Chicken, Turkey - 2 to 3 hours.

Heavy nuts like Almonds, peanuts, cashew, walnut, and pecan - up to 3 hours.

Milk and low fat dairy takes up to 90 minutes while heavy fat dairy like butter and cheese can take up to 5 hours.

Beef, lamb - 3 to 4.

Pork – 4 to 5 hours.

Chapter 11 - External Information.

If you bought my book, you are welcome to join in our discussion groups and even e-mail me directly with any questions.

To lose weight is definitely not an easy task. For those of us who saw the sizes going relentlessly up over long periods of time, it is even more difficult. Please join our groups – it is absolutely free. Or you can join others. It does not really matter to me, my only wish is that many people will find this book a motivation to start walking the road to a thinner, lighter and much healthier body.

My personal eMail is: corrielamprecht@outlook.com – but do not spam me, I will block and report you.

My Facebook Page, especially for this book is:

https://www.facebook.com/Book.Obese

And for my other books you can see Facebook at:

https://www.facebook.com/corrie.ebooks

My Book Writing website is: http://www.corrie-books.com and from there you can go to the Books menu, follow links to this book page where you will also find additional information and links to other people's pages, videos and studies.

That page will be continuously updated.

Dear Reader,

I hope you have enjoyed this book and above all, that you find it of value.

The bookstore where you bought the book (or my website) has a feature for customers to post a review. All such product reviews are important to the author, the marketplace and other potential customers.

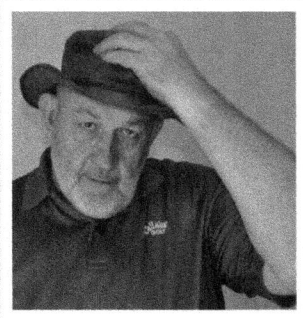

Could I kindly ask from you this very big favour.

Would you spare a minute and write a review for me. Please?

We do appreciate all reviews, positive and negative. I trust that if you are not happy with this product, you will give me some constructive comments included in your review. If you are reasonably happy, it is a great motivation for me as writer to continue on this tenuous path.

I will try to post a direct link to this book's page and also to my Authors Page if that is available. You might be lucky to just click on the link below – else you need to go through your normal log-in.

In gratitude.

Corrie Lamprecht

www.ingramcontent.com/pod-product-compliance
Lightning Source LLC
Chambersburg PA
CBHW062207280526
45788CB00001B/486